Integrated Anatomy

Contents

Preface

Anatomy has been, and remains, a core discipline within clinical practice. It provides the basic language and understanding of the human body essential for sound clinical examination and practice. There has been an increasing emphasis within education for learning within context, coupled with a reduction in classroom time for students. Today anatomy teaching is frequently integrated with other disciplines and taught using a systems approach rather than the traditional regional approach.

This text aims to provide the anatomical background for the undergraduate medical student to understand clinical practice prior to specialisation. It would be useful for practitioners involved in introducing students to clinical practice. This book will also be useful to both those in training and in postgraduate study, and to students in the professions allied to medicine, especially radiographers.

The authors have selected anatomical detail to produce a comprehensive and clinically relevant primer gross anatomy text, presented using a regional approach. However, to assist the student on a systems course, within each region, information has been presented by system. Embryology and many short clinical scenarios have been woven throughout to illustrate how the anatomy presents in, or influences, clinical practice. The book is illustrated throughout with clinical, anatomical and radiological figures, drawings and photographs. The radiological imaging helps the reader to relate gross anatomy learning to images that will be seen in the clinical situation.

The approach used should help the reader to put core anatomical knowledge within a clinical context and hence provide a firm basis to practise as a doctor to the benefit of our patients.

D. Heylings
R. Spence
B. Kelly

Cardiac muscle is not connected to the skeleton, though it does work on its own internal fibrous skeleton that forms the anchor point for the one-way valves and for the muscle fibres to contract against. Each side of the heart, the right and left, are basically the same. There is a receiving chamber, or atrium, into which the veins drain. On contraction of the atria, blood passes into the corresponding ventricle through the atrioventricular valve, whose cusps are tethered to mounds of ventricular muscle, papillary muscles. When the ventricles contract the atrioventricular valves close and blood is forced into the main exit arteries through semilunar valves. These valves normally consist of three cup-like cusps. When the ventricles relax, the elastic recoil of the artery pushes blood into the cusps, filling them and hence closing the valves.

Blood passes from the right ventricle to the lungs before being returned to the left side of the heart from where it is pumped into the aorta for distribution by the left side of the heart (Fig. 1.7).

RESPIRATORY SYSTEM

This system allows the body to absorb the vital oxygen directly into the blood stream and exchange it for waste carbon dioxide. It consists of an opening (the nares) located on the face opening into a right and left nasal cavity. Within the cavity the surface area is greatly increased by three turbinates (conchae) attached to the lateral walls. The resultant large surface area is able to moisten and warm the incoming air and larger foreign particles are prevented from going further into the body. Warmed air then passes into the

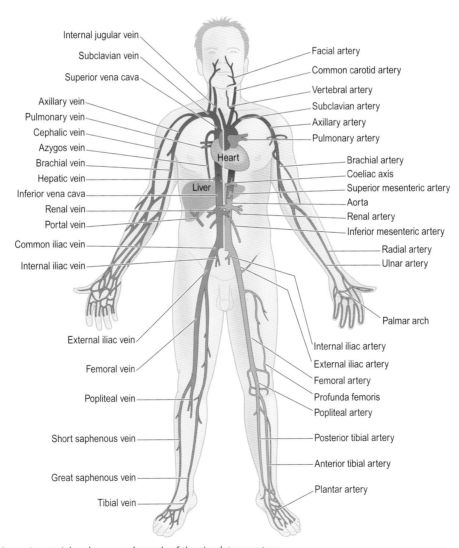

Fig. 1.7 Overview of the main arterial and venous channels of the circulatory system.

common space posterior to the nasal cavities, the nasopharynx superior to the palate, and descends into the common area for both the respiratory and gastrointestinal systems, the oropharynx. It then continues into the laryngeal part of the laryngopharynx and hence through the vocal cords into the trachea, then through the bronchi into the lungs to be distributed through ever decreasing bronchi and bronchioles before finally terminating in the alveoli, the delicate air sacs (Fig. 1.8) where the gas exchange takes place.

Surrounding each nasal cavity is a series of air sinuses (frontal, maxillary, sphenoidal, ethmoidal) within the bones of the face and skull. These lighten the facial skeleton and provide an increased area to moisten air and provide an increased resonance to the voice. Within the nasal cavity, the epithelium at the opening of the nasal cavity is hairy, stratified, squamous and keratinised, marking a continuation of the surface of the skin, in addition to which the concentration of hairs is able to filter out large particles.

On proceeding into the nasal cavity past the squamous epithelium, the cavity becomes lined by pseudostratified ciliated columnar epithelium, which contains many goblet cells (Fig. 1.8). This epithelium is the basic type seen through-out the upper airways of the nasal cavities, the nasopharynx and inferiorly from the opening to the larynx to the trachea and into the bronchi. In the alveoli the epithelium is very thin, giving a blood/air barrier of approximately 0.3 μm. However, it is important to remember that the epithelium covering the vocal cords is stratified squamous non-keratinising epithelium, reflecting the function of the vocal cords. The mucosa in the nasal cavity is very vascular to warm the incoming air. If the vessels underlying the mucosa dilate, the mucosa can swell up considerably, reducing the space within the cavity for normal airflow and giving the individual a feeling of a blocked nose. The mucus produced by the mucosa traps larger particles, which the cilia move posteriorly into the oral part of the pharynx, where they can be swallowed. Within the larynx and bronchi, the cilia move the mucus (now trapping the finer particles) upwards towards the laryngopharynx where it can pass into the pharynx and hence be swallowed.

As potentially harmful particles, including microbes, are carried in the air, there is a ring of lymphoid tissue located in the naso- and oropharynx designed to ensure a rapid response to potential pathogens.

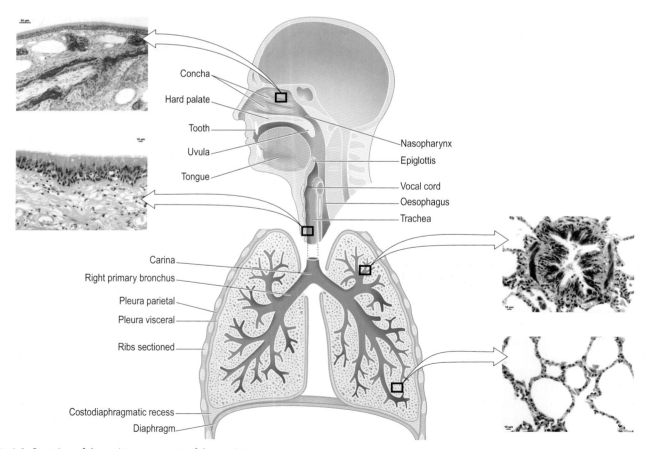

Fig. 1.8 Overview of the main components of the respiratory system; inserts are histological sections demonstrating the mucosal structure at 50 μm (stain H & E, courtesy of Stephen McCullough, Queen's University, Belfast).

Table 1.1 SUMMARY OF RADIOLOGICAL TERMS

MODALITY	'BRIGHTNESS' (FINAL IMAGE WHITER)	'DARKNESS' (FINAL IMAGE DARKER)
Plain X-ray	Density (more solid)	Lucency (less dense)
Ultrasound	Hyperechoic (reflects sound)	Hypoechoic (transmits sound)
CT	High attenuation	Low attenuation
MRI	High signal	Low signal
Nuclear medicine	Focus of high activity	Photopenic

Today, when reviewing radiological or nuclear medicine studies, we typically infer conclusions from the images produced on a screen or on photographic film. These images are composed of shades of grey ranging from white to black. On some studies, e.g. plain radiographs, only 4 densities or shades can be distinguished: bone (white), soft tissue (grey), fat (a darker grey) and air (black). In contrast, computerised tomography (CT) uses thousands of grey shades.

The different branches of imaging use different terminologies to describe these greyscales; however, Table 1.1 summarises the accepted terminologies.

Orientation

As in anatomy, radiological images are viewed in standard orientations. In recent years CT and magnetic resonance imaging (MRI) development has greatly increased the possible orientations that the final image can be reconstructed, using a process known as multiplanar reformatting (MPR). However, conventions still apply based on the traditional anatomical planes (see Fig. 1.1):

- Sagittal images show a slice (projection) through the long axis from anterior to posterior.
- Coronal images show a slice through the long axis from the right side to left side.
- Axial (transverse or horizontal) images show a horizontal slice at right angles to the long axis of the body. These images are normally viewed as if standing at a patient's feet looking up towards their head.

Reviewing radiographs

Although a comprehensive review of imaging is beyond the scope of this book, there are some general considerations when interpreting radiographs. First, ensure that the patient details are correct, i.e. patient name, unit number and the date of the examination. Next, evaluate each image in a systematic way, using 'review areas', e.g. on a chest radiograph, look at the heart, the pulmonary vessels, the lung fields, the bony skeleton and the diaphragm. By viewing the image in a structured way, the viewer is *less* likely to miss abnormalities.

The chest radiograph (Fig. 4.2)

Review:

- In the mediastinal shadow (the dense area in the middle of the image).
  - Is the heart of normal size (less than half the width of the chest) or enlarged (greater than half the width of the chest)? Is its silhouette normal?
  - Is there the normal outline of the aortic arch and the hilar vessels (passing into the lucent areas to the sides)? The latter should be of the same size, and density. At the top of the image is the trachea central (a lucent track normally in the midline) or is it displaced?
- The lung fields (the lucent or dark areas on either side of the mediastinum). The pulmonary vessels should not be visible in the outer third of the lungs (if they are, this indicates heart failure). Look for focal masses and infections (shown as areas of increased density). A visible lung edge suggests pneumothorax – check for tracheal displacement to the other side, i.e. away from the pneumothorax.
- The bony skeleton. Check the ribs for fractures and malignant destruction. Are the shoulder joints normal? Is there any evidence of joint dislocation, arthritis, or fracture?
- The diaphragm (inferiorly). Is there free air under it within the abdominal cavity? Check the recess where it meets the rib cage. If not clearly seen, there could be a pleural effusion (fluid within the pleural cavity).

Postero-anterior and antero-posterior chest radiographs

With a postero-anterior (PA) chest radiograph, the patient stands with their anterior chest wall against the imaging plate, and the X-ray tube behind them (at a distance of 180 cm). With an antero-posterior (AP) film, the film cassette is placed behind the patient. Typically, as AP films are performed in bed-bound patients, the cassette is between the patient and their pillow. The tube is in front of the patient. For both studies, the image is acquired on maximal inspiration. The convention is that a chest radiograph which is not PA will have its method of acquisition abbreviated on it, e.g. 'AP; Semi-erect, Supine'.

Advantages of PA chest radiograph:

1. Scapulae move laterally, and the clavicles upwards, giving greater visualisation of the lung fields.
2. The dose to the thyroid and breast is reduced
3. The heart and mediastinum lie closer to the imaging plate, and therefore are less magnified.

The abdominal radiograph (Fig. 6.2)

Review:

- The bowel gas pattern. Is there gaseous dilatation of the small and/or large bowel (usually there is little gas in the small or large bowel)? This may indicate intestinal obstruction. Check the pelvis. Is there gas within the pelvis in the rectum? Its presence excludes acute obstruction of the bowel.

- Are there abnormal gas collections outside the bowel, e.g. under the diaphragm? If present these may indicate an abscess or free air (pneumoperitoneum) due to organ perforation or surgical intervention.
- Bones. Evaluate the lumbar spine for normal alignment, fractures, and arthritis. Check the pedicles are present. An absent pedicle is a sign of malignant bony infiltration. Review the pelvic bones for fractures, arthritic changes and maglinant destruction.
- Soft tissues. The liver, spleen and kidney outlines may be visible. Check for organ enlargement. Look at the shadows of the two psoas muscles.
- Calcifications. Gallstones and renal calculi may be seen. Arterial calcification can be seen, in particular aortic calcification and if curved, should suggest aortic aneurysm – a potentially fatal condition.
- Artefacts. Surgical clips, aortic, renal and biliary stents, and intrauterine contraceptive devices are commonly seen artefacts.

The skeletal radiograph

There are some general principles:

1. Bone radiographs should include the joint at either end, e.g. radiographs of the humerus should also include the shoulder and elbow joints. Bone contours are usually smooth. Fractures are often associated with joint dislocations.

2. Bone and joint radiographs typically require two views at right angles to each other (orthogonal views), usually anterior and lateral projections, as an injury, although very obvious on one view, can be subtle on the other! Again check bone contours looking for irregularities.

3. Look carefully at the surrounding soft tissues. Fluid collections near joints (effusions) are significant, Foreign body artefacts, such as glass fragments or shrapnel, may suggest more serious injury.

Contrast media

Because of the diverse nature of the many imaging modalities currently available, the mode of action of the many contrast media is necessarily diverse and complex. There are, fortunately, some common facts. Contrast media have two functions:

1. The delineation of normal structures (e.g. the gastrointestinal tract, biliary tree, thecal sac, joint spaces and blood vessels).

2. Improved visibility between a focal mass and the surrounding organ parenchyma. This is commonly known as 'lesion enhancement'.

Essentially, radiological contrast agents accentuate a structure or abnormality by increasing its visibility against its background. Examples include a mass in the liver, a stricture in the bowel or blood vessel, or a renal calculus (stone) blocking an obstructed contrast-filled ureter. These images can be enhanced digitally by subtracting one part of the image to enhance other structures of interest, a process known as digital subtraction.

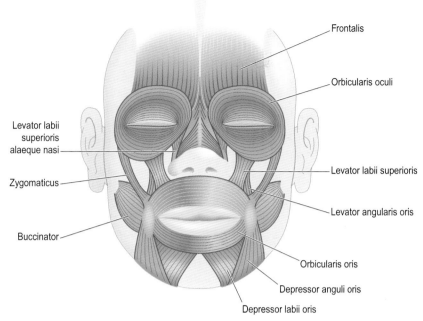

Fig. 2.12 Superficial muscles of facial expression (innervated by the 7th cranial nerve).

oris) and one around each eye socket (orbicularis oculi). In life these are used to reduce the size of the enclosed opening, puckering of the lips and screwing the eyes tightly closed. Attached to each side of the oral cavity is an elevator (levator angularis oris) and a depressor (depressor angularis oris). The nasal cavity also has levators designed to widen the soft nasal openings.

Clinically the role of these muscles is clearly demonstrated when the nerve supply, the facial nerve, is disrupted. In such a case, the affected side of the face becomes smooth, the wrinkles vanish and when talking or smiling the face twists towards the normal unaffected side. It is worth noting that paralysis of orbicularis oculi exposes the cornea and it is in danger of ulceration. Two muscles within this sheet of facial muscles lie within the scalp, frontalis lying anteriorly and occipitalis posteriorly. Contraction of these muscles tenses the aponeurosis of the scalp and anteriorly creates transverse creases on the forehead. In a process to flatten the wrinkles of the forehead, plastic surgeons inject this latter muscle with the botulism toxin to paralyse the muscle (often referred to as 'Botox' injections).

Muscles of mastication

The muscles of mastication are designed to move the mandible and assist in the initiation of digestion. These muscles are powerful, in particular those closing the mandible to cut the food. Then the other muscles come into play moving the mandible from side to side as the food is ground between the molar teeth before swallowing. Temporalis (Fig. 2.13) is a large fan-shaped muscle attaching to the lateral aspect of the

parietal, frontal and squamous part of the temporal bones. Anteriorly it attaches to the zygoma medial to the zygomatic arch. From this broad attachment the muscle fibres descend to attach to the coronoid process and to the anteromedial aspect of the mandible and in action it is a powerful closer of the jaw.

The masseter passes inferiorly from the zygomatic arch to attach to the lateral aspect of the ramus of the mandible. Like temporalis, the masseter is a powerful closer of the jaw. The lateral pterygoid plate provides the medial attachment for the smaller lateral pterygoid muscle (Fig. 2.13), which joins a superior head attaching to the adjacent base of the skull before passing laterally to attach to the condylar fossa, anterior to the condyle of the mandible. Superiorly the fibres of this muscle also attach to the anterior aspect of the capsule of the temporomandibular joint and hence to the fibrous disc which is itself firmly adherent to the inside of the capsule. Finally the medial pterygoid muscle, attaching to the fossa between the medial and lateral pterygoid plates, passes laterally and inferiorly to attach to the medial aspect of the angle of the mandible inferior to the mandibular foramen. Both pterygoid muscles are responsible, when working unilaterally, for moving the jaw from side to side as in grinding. There has been considerable discussion concerning how precisely lateral pterygoid comes into play as it is also able to pull the temporomandibular disc anteriorly, when opening the mouth, as the mandibular condyle glides forwards. The mandibular branch of the trigeminal nerve supplies these four muscles of mastication.

In addition to these four muscles of mastication there is a fifth muscle, **buccinator** (Fig. 2.13), without which an

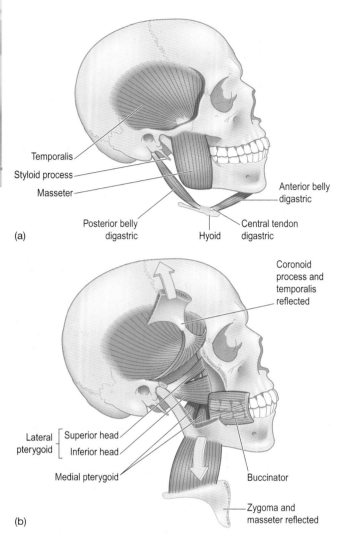

(a)

(b)

Fig. 2.13 Muscles of mastication: (a) superficial – temporalis, masseter, digastric; (b) deep – lateral, medial pterygoid muscles.

individual has difficulty in maintaining the food between the teeth. This muscle forms the cheek, attaching on each side lateral to the teeth, superiorly to the maxilla and inferiorly to the mandible. Anteriorly it has a free edge but posteriorly it attaches to the pterygomandibular raphe to which the superior constrictor attaches (see below). Unlike the other muscles of mastication this muscle is innervated, along with the muscles of facial expression, by the facial nerve. When testing the facial nerve, if the facial nerve is damaged, the patient will be unable to suck in the affected cheek, or whistle, and food will collect between the affected cheek and teeth on the same side.

Superficially in the neck is platysma, a thin sheet of muscle just deep to the skin. It passes inferiorly from the mandible to the skin of the upper thorax. Deep to platysma in the anterior neck are the strap muscles passing superiorly from the sternum to the thyroid cartilage and the hyoid bone (Fig. 2.14). The function of this group is to depress the thyroid cartilage and hyoid bone. In effect they act as the inferior group of fixators for these structures. In particular, by fixing the hyoid it provides a base for the muscles of the tongue and floor of the mouth to act (see below).

Superior to the hyoid are the two digastric muscles (Figs. 2.13, 2.14). Together they act as elevators of the hyoid and act in opposition to the strap muscles when fixing the hyoid bone. Each digastric muscle has a posterior and an anterior belly, with the central tendon tethered to the hyoid. Anteriorly digastric attaches to the mandible whilst posteriorly it attaches to the mastoid process. Deep to digastric lies another elevator of the hyoid, a flat sheet of muscle, mylohyoid. This muscle passes from the anterolateral aspect of the mandible inferiorly to the superior aspect of the hyoid. Working alone it will elevate the hyoid, or acting with

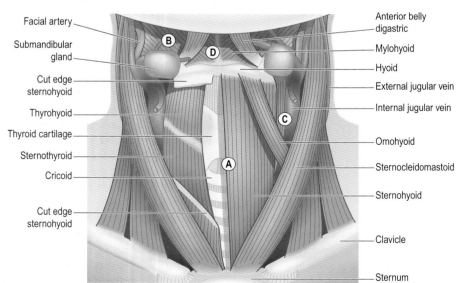

Fig. 2.14 Muscles of the anterior triangle of the neck: A, muscle triangle; B, digastric triangle; C, carotid triangle; D, submental triangle.

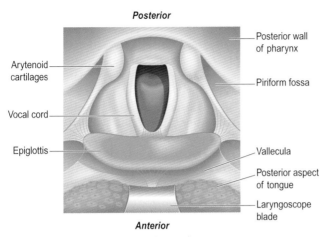

Posterior

Arytenoid cartilages

Vocal cord

Epiglottis

Posterior wall of pharynx

Piriform fossa

Vallecula

Posterior aspect of tongue

Laryngoscope blade

Anterior

Fig. 2.26 View of larynx as seen down a laryngoscope.

bone for the upper third. It is lined medially with the same respiratory mucosa (mucus-secreting) as the nasopharynx and with ciliated columnar epithelium nearer the tympanic (middle ear) cavity. In the nasopharynx the opening of the auditory tube is slit-like and normally closed except when swallowing or yawning, when it opens. It is surrounded by lymphoid tissue (tubal tonsil). The auditory tube provides a mechanism to allow the pressure within the ear to equalise with that of the surrounding atmosphere. In the presence of upper respiratory tract infections the auditory tube may become blocked. In such a case the air in the middle ear is absorbed and 'ear' pain may result from the negative pressure within the middle ear cavity compared to the surrounding atmosphere. Alternatively the infection can travel along the auditory tube and infect the middle ear with a resultant accumulation of fluid.

LYMPHATIC (IMMUNE) SYSTEM

A 77-year-old woman came to her doctor with a swelling in the left posterior triangle of her neck. The swelling felt very hard and her doctor was concerned that this represented an enlarged lymph node containing a secondary carcinoma. On referral to hospital the examining physician also felt the lymph node was enlarged and was concerned.

A needle biopsy was performed but did not give a complete answer and therefore an open excision biopsy was required. This was undertaken under anaesthetic. Following surgery the patient complained that she was unable to elevate her arm to brush her hair on that side. When the surgeon examined her after the operation he found that she had a paralysis of trapezius muscle on the side of the surgery and hence her inability to elevate the shoulder and arm above 90°. It was then clear that the surgeon had inadvertently removed a section of the accessory nerve as it traversed

the posterior triangle (see above). The movement of the sternocleidomastoid muscle on that side, also supplied by the accessory nerve, was intact as its motor branch was given off from the accessory nerve as it traversed anterior to the internal jugular vein before entering the posterior triangle of the neck.

The node pathology confirmed secondary carcinoma from a primary lung tumour and the patient required chemotherapy. The nerve did not recover and for the rest of her short life the patient had difficulty in brushing her hair due to the absence of an active trapezius muscle on that side.

There is a ring of lymph nodes around the base of the skull and inferior to the mandible. Lymphatic channels drain the face and scalp to the nearest group of nodes. The back of the scalp drains to the **occipital nodes** (posteriorly) and the **mastoid nodes** laterally (Fig. 2.27). The infratemporal fossa and lateral orbit drain to nodes around and within the parotid gland, **parotid nodes**. The medial aspect of the orbit, the anterior face and oral cavity all drain to the **submandibular group** of lymph nodes, lying inferior to the mandible, while the central portion of the lower lip drains to the **submental group** of nodes. Inferiorly these nodes drain to the **deep lymphatic chain** located along the carotid sheath and lie deep to sternocleidomastoid. On reaching the root of the neck this channel drains into the brachiocephalic vein on the right and on the left, either into the thoracic duct or directly into either the caudal aspect of the internal jugular vein or the subclavian vein. In addition to the nodes lying superficial to sternocleidomastoid, there are a few **superficial cervical nodes** located more posteriorly in the upper aspect

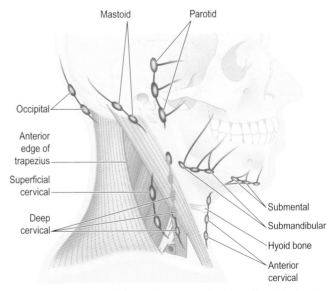

Mastoid

Parotid

Occipital

Anterior edge of trapezius

Superficial cervical

Deep cervical

Submental

Submandibular

Hyoid bone

Anterior cervical

Fig. 2.27 Distribution of the main groups of lymph nodes of the head and neck.

of the posterior triangle of the neck to which the occipital nodes drain first. These are related to the accessory nerve (see case above). The childhood infection mumps involves enlargement of the parotid group of nodes in particular, giving the child the classic appearance of a unilateral (or bilateral) swollen cheek.

Another ring of lymphoid tissue, Waldeyer's ring, exists within the head and neck, at the junction of the nasopharynx superiorly, with the oropharynx inferiorly and the oral cavity anteriorly. It consists of (a) the nasopharyngeal tonsil, often referred to as 'the adenoids', lying superior to the soft palate in the posterior wall, (b) the palatine tonsil, inferior to the palate lying posterolaterally in the oral cavity between the palatoglossal and palatopharyngeal folds, and (c) the lingual tonsil seen as collections of lymphoid tissue on the dorsum of the posterior aspect of the tongue.

GASTROINTESTINAL SYSTEM

The oral cavity marks the start of the gastrointestinal system. The lips are formed from orbicularis oris, the elevators and depressors of the angle of the mouth. Laterally buccinator forms the cheeks. Superiorly is the hard and soft palates separating the oral cavity from the nasal cavity.

Embryology

A baby boy was born and immediately the parents noticed that he had a defect in his lip just below the nose. On closer inspection of his mouth the palate appeared also to be split in the midline.

The baby underwent immediate corrective surgery to repair his lip. The baby was unable to feed properly because of the gap in his palate and this was closed temporarily by a prosthesis while the baby grew. This allowed the child to feed.

At the age of 2 years the gap in the palate was closed surgically. Unfortunately this was only partially successful and the patient required speech therapy as he grew older because of a persistent lisp and nasal speech.

The face arises from three components, namely left and right **maxillary processes**, right and left **mandibular processes** and a single **frontonasal process**. Inferiorly (caudally) the mandibular processes grow to fuse together in the midline, forming the mandible inferior to the buccal opening or future mouth (Fig. 2.28). Likewise the two maxillary processes will eventually fuse with the frontonasal process to form the bony structures superior to the buccal opening.

Two small thickenings of ectoderm then appear in the frontonasal process and these deepen to form the nasal pits.

Ridges medial and lateral to the pits enlarge and the two medial ridges fuse to form the primitive nose. The pits deepen and grow to form a large cavity within the nose, the future nasal cavity. Laterally, the maxillary processes grow larger and become fused to the lateral margins of the frontonasal process, giving rise to the future cheeks. The eye develops superior to this process and the lacrimal duct develops along the fusion line of the two processes. The medial part of the lower border of the maxillary process forms the lateral components of upper lips. At the same time the frontonasal process in the midline forms the philtrum (Fig. 2.28) and adjacent midline component of the upper lip. On the oral aspect of this process it contributes to the formation of the small triangular-shaped primary palate, from which later arise the upper incisor teeth. Lateral plates of tissue, initially angled inferiorly, form along the lateral aspects of the developing mouth from the maxillary process to form palatine processes. However, as the tongue forms, the palatine processes are pushed upwards (elevated). As a result they are able to grow medially and eventually fuse with each other and the primary palate along the midline. Thus the upper border of the oral cavity is formed, giving rise in time to the hard and soft palates and the uvula. Failure of fusion of the palatine palates can lead to a cleft palate. Similarly, failure of fusion of the maxillary process and frontonasal process can lead to a unilateral cleft lip being present, which can be bilateral if both processes are affected.

Oral cavity

Dominant within the oral cavity are the two rows of teeth and the tongue attached to the floor of the mouth. Between the lips and teeth is the smaller space within the oral cavity, the vestibule, whilst the main part of the oral cavity lies between the teeth and contains the tongue. In the adult there are 32 teeth in total. In each half of the jaw (Figs. 2.8, 2.17) from the lips posteriorly are two incisors, a canine, two premolars and three molar teeth, the most posterior of which is known as the 'wisdom' tooth, erupting as it does after 18 years. It is the crown of the tooth that is visible above the gums with the root buried within the bone of the jaw (Fig. 2.29). The incisors with a flattened upper surface are designed to cut, the pointy canines are for tearing, whilst the premolar and molar teeth with their flattened upper surface are designed to grind and chew. In the young child (less than 6 years) dentition consists of a set of 20 deciduous teeth, two incisors, a canine and two molar teeth in each half of upper and lower jaws. These will be lost as the permanent dentition starts to erupt from the sixth year of life.

Arising from the floor of the mouth is the tongue with its roughened superior surface containing the taste buds laterally in the **fungiform papillae**. As with the rest of the oral cavity, the mucosa of the tongue is stratified squamous in type. Inferior to the tongue in the midline is the frenulum,

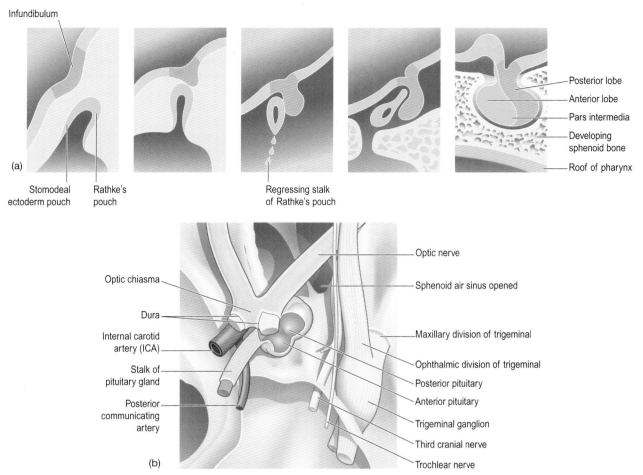

Fig. 2.37 The pituitary gland: (a) development (from Larsen 2001 Human Embryology 3rd Edn. Churchill Livingstone, Philadelphia, with permission), (b) in situ. The surrounding bone and structures on the right of the gland have been removed for clarity.

CSF in the subarachnoid space, the arachnoid mater lies against the deep surface of the outermost meningeal layer, the **dura mater**, separated from it by the potential subdural space. The dura of the cranial cavity consists of fibrous tissue which, within the cranial cavity, is normally firmly adherent to the more superficial periosteum (**endosteum**) of the inner skull. There is no extra- (epi-) dural space within the cranium, only a potential space within which lies the middle meningeal artery providing an arterial supply to the cranial dura. The dura within the cranial cavity is continuous with the dura of the spinal canal through the foramen magnum. However, the dura in the vertebral canal does not attach to the surrounding bone and so maintains an extra- (epi-) dural space.

The dura forms several important folds that help to divide the cranial cavity (Fig. 2.24). These folds consist of a double layer of dura. In the sagittal plane there is a longitudinal fold passing posteriorly between the two cerebral hemispheres, the **falx cerebri**, which is larger posteriorly than anteriorly. It is secured anteriorly to the **crista galli**, the vertical plate of the ethmoid bone. Posteriorly the falx blends with another fold of dura, the **tentorium cerebelli**. This fold lies in the transverse plane passing from the superior edge of the petrous temporal bone anteriorly and in the same plane as the internal occipital protuberance posteriorly.

A 9-year-old boy was brought by his mother to the A&E department with an 18-hour history of pyrexia and vomiting. When he was seen by the paediatric doctor, the child complained that the lights in the examination cubicle were hurting his eyes (photophobia). He was noted to have a stiff and painful neck. There were no other clinical findings, in particular there were no neurological signs and no evidence of raised intracranial pressure. The doctor also noted that there was no rash. Despite this last negative finding, a provisional diagnosis of meningitis was made. A lumbar puncture was performed and specimen of CSF sent for bacteriology and biochemistry. A blood sample confirmed the white cell count was elevated.

The patient was commenced on intravenous broad-spectrum antibiotics immediately following the lumbar puncture.

Intravenous fluids were also given. CSF subsequently did confirm bacterial meningitis. Because meningitis is a 'notifiable disease', the Department of Public Health was informed and antibiotic prophylaxis was arranged for the boy's family and close contacts. The boy subsequently made a full recovery.

Many of the intracranial venous sinuses lie in an endothelial lined space between the periosteum superficially and the deeper fibrous dura (Figs. 2.2, 2.24). However, the inferior sagittal sinus and the straight sinus lie between two layers of the fibrous dura as they are not related to underlying bone. Venous channels draining the cerebral hemispheres cross between the cerebral surface and the superior sagittal sinus. These channels cross both the subarachnoid and subdural spaces to drain directly into the sagittal venous sinus itself. The brain is 'mobile' within the fluid-filled cranial cavity, and these venous channels act as a means of tethering the brain, so limiting its ability to move.

Cerebrospinal fluid

The cerebrospinal fluid is filtered from the blood within spaces (ventricles) in the cerebral tissue (Fig. 2.38), from thin vascular tissue, the **choroid plexus**. Most of the CSF is produced in the two lateral ventricles, though the choroid plexus in the third and fourth ventricles produces some more. There is a circulation pattern within the brain from the lateral ventricles into the midline third ventricle, through the narrow cerebral aqueduct in the midbrain into the midline fourth ventricle. From here CSF flows out through a lateral recess into the subarachnoid space where it flows down around the spinal cord and upwards around the

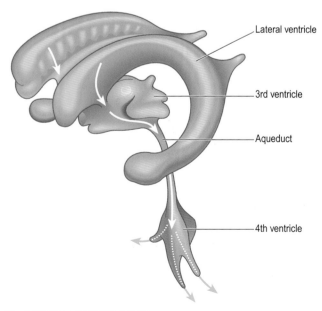

Lateral ventricle

3rd ventricle

Aqueduct

4th ventricle

Fig. 2.38 The ventricular system.

cerebral hemispheres. It is finally absorbed and passed back into the venous system through grape-like extensions of the arachnoid mater that lie within the superior sagittal sinus, the **arachnoid granulations**. Blockage of the circulation pathways will result in an increase of pressure within the system proximal to the blockage, producing a condition known as hydrocephalus.

The first evidence of the development of the central nervous system (CNS) appears around the middle of the third week. A dorsal thickening of ectoderm termed the **neural plate** is induced by the signal agents from the notochord and paraxial mesoderm and becomes infolded to form an axial groove. This is the **neural groove**, with neural folds on each side. During the fourth week, the neural folds fuse together to form the **neural tube**. Some cells at the apex of the neural folds form a separate cell mass termed the **neural crest** and these develop into components of the autonomic nervous system as well as a number of other tissues, including Schwann cells and the adrenal medulla. A central lumen is present in the neural tube and this forms the neural canal, which in turn develops into the ventricles of the brain and the central canal of the spinal cord. Abnormalities within the development here can lead to abnormal CSF flow, e.g. blockage of the cerebral aqueduct, and can lead to hydrocephalus which if undetected can lead to severe damage to the developing brain of the neonate.

A 9-year-old boy was brought to his GP by his parents who noted that he was having difficulty with his balance and was complaining of headaches. He also had had several episodes of urinary incontinence and his teachers had complained about his recent progress at school. The GP noted that his head circumference was on the 95th centile having previously measured on the 60th centile at his most recent attendance and that the tone in his legs was increased.

He was referred to the neurosurgical unit at the local teaching hospital and a CT scan was performed. This showed the presence of dilated lateral and third ventricles with a normal fourth ventricle. There was effacement of the overlying cortical sulci in the brain and a diagnosis of hydrocephalus was made and an MRI was recommended. This showed that the cerebral aqueduct (of Sylvius) was stenosed. The boy subsequently had a third ventriculostomy performed in which a small hole is made that allows communication between the floor of the third ventricle and the suprasellar cistern. His symptoms resolved rapidly.

In the very young child with hydrocephalus, the cranial cavity has the ability to enlarge considerably as the bones of the skull vault are able to move apart compensating for the increasing pressure within the cranial cavity, maintaining a relatively normal intracranial pressure. However, as the skull matures and the fontanelles close, the raised intracranial pressure damages the cerebral tissue and the child tracts (spinocerebellar) passing from these nuclei to the cerebellum. On each side of midline, throughout the medulla and the pons, the important cranial nerve nuclei are located. In the upper third of the medulla lies the **solitary tract** with its surrounding nuclei involved in mediating taste.

An old part of the brain, known as the **limbic system**, consists of (a) the cingulate gyrus, just superior to the corpus callosum, extending posteriorly into the parahippocampal gyrus of the temporal lobe, (b) the mamillary bodies and (c) the hypothalamus and is connected to the olfactory mechanism. Function is complex and is involved in maintaining homeostasis, body temperature, emotion, eating behaviour, sexual behaviour and gonadal regulation, and its action is exerted through the effects of the hypothalamus and pituitary gland.

Cranial nerves

The **twelve cranial nerves** leave the surface of the brain to innervate the structures primarily of the head but also of the neck and trunk. These nerves are numbered from anterior to posterior as they leave the surface of the brain. The central nuclei of ten of these twelve important nerves are located in the midbrain and the hindbrain, the exceptions being the first and second cranial nerves.

On the inferior aspect of the frontal lobes of the cerebral hemispheres is a tract of nervous tissue known as the **olfactory tract**. Passing anteriorly it swells to form the olfactory bulb superior to the cribriform plate of the ethmoid bone. It is from the olfactory bulb that about 20 short **olfactory (first cranial) nerves** descend from their cell bodies and pass through the holes in the **cribriform plate** directly into the specialised ciliated epithelium in the superior aspect of the nasal cavity. Posteriorly the olfactory tract passes into the substance of the brain lateral to the optic chiasma (see below) and continues laterally to terminate in the main olfactory cortex located in the uncus of the temporal lobe (Fig. 2.39). These axons do not pass to the thalamus but to parts of the limbic system. Following a severe blow to the front of the skull, it is possible that a patient may sustain a fracture through the delicate ethmoid bone. In the presence of such a fracture, the patient may complain of a diminution of smell, food being less tasty and a clear fluid discharge from the nares. The fluid discharge should be tested for sugar and, if rich in sugar, is indicative of a CSF leak.

Visible on the inferior surface of the frontal lobe is the **chiasma** of the optic tract, seen as an 'X' just posterior to the olfactory tract and anterior to the pituitary stalk, from which the two **optic (second cranial) nerves** pass anterolaterally. They pass through the optic canal (in the body of the sphenoid bone, Fig. 2.7) as the optic nerve to enter the orbit and pass through the ring of posterior attachments of the extrinsic eye muscles. On reaching the posterior aspect of the globe of the eye, it passes through the sclera at an area visualised inside the eye as the **optic disc** or blind spot. At this point within the eye the axons spread out across the surface of the retina to their cell bodies, the ganglion cells. These cells are stimulated by light triggering a response from the visual cells, the **rods** and **cones**, lying in contact with the pigmented layer via a bipolar cell (see Fig. 2.50).

To reach the rods and cones, light has to pass through the retinal layer containing the ganglion cells and their axons. Then light passes through the bipolar layer, triggering the visual response before being absorbed by the pigmented layer. Images received on the retina of each eye pass into the nerve so that those from the medial or nasal retina lie on the medial aspect of the optic nerve, whilst those from the lateral or temporal retina lie on the lateral aspect. Damage to the optic nerve will result in blindness within that eye. On reaching the optic chiasma (superior to the pituitary fossa) the nasal nerve fibres cross to the opposite side of the midline. Posterior to the chiasma, the *optic nerve* is now referred to as the *optic tract* and passes posterolaterally to the **lateral geniculate nucleus** of the thalamus. After relaying (synapsing) in this nucleus, the *optic radiation* passes posteriorly to the visual cortex in the occipital pole of the cerebral hemisphere superior to the tentorium cerebelli. Damage to the optic tract and radiation will result in the loss of visual field to one side of midline (homonymous hemianopia). However, damage to the occipital cortex itself, as might result from falling backwards and hitting the occiput on the ground, will result in bilateral central loss of visual field (a scotoma). Crossing of the nasal retinal axons in the chiasma means that the left cerebral cortex receives images that lie to the right of the nose (temporal retina of left eye and nasal retina on a right eye) and the right visual cortex sees images of objects located to the left side of the nose. Enlargement of the pituitary gland can damage the nasal fibres crossing in the chiasma (see case on page 47). As a result the patient loses peripheral vision in both eyes (tunnel vision). Some visual fibres leave the optic tract before the lateral geniculate nucleus to reach the superior colliculus of the midbrain and are involved in the pupillary light reflex mediated through the third cranial nerve.

A 57-year-old man presented to his general practitioner complaining of headache, poor concentration and blurred vision getting worse over 6 months. On direct questioning by his doctor he said the headaches were mild and not associated with any specific symptoms such as vomiting or photophobia. The visual disturbance was described as 'darkness on the right side' and had been causing difficulties with driving. The patient's wife, who was present at the consultation, reported that he was becoming more irritable and also forgetful. The patient's past medical history was unremarkable.

On examination the doctor observed a loss of the patient's visual field to the right (homonymous hemianopia). The remainder of the examination was normal and he was referred for a CT scan. This revealed a large mass arising from the left skull base close to the pituitary fossa (Fig. 2.46). It had an area of high density, which contained some calcification, and another area of low density within the surrounding brain due to the pressure from the tumour. These findings were consistent with a meningioma, a slow-growing benign brain tumour.

Tumour

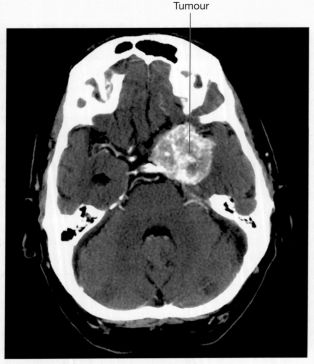

Fig. 2.46 CT image of a left-sided (parasellar) meningioma in the region of the pituitary stalk.

Passing forwards through the substance of the midbrain from the oculomotor nucleus (lying just anterior to the aqueduct), the **oculomotor (third cranial) nerve** leaves the anterior aspect of the midbrain (Fig. 2.39). This nerve pierces the dura at the posterolateral aspect of the cavernous sinus to continue anteriorly in its lateral wall to leave the cranial cavity through the superior orbital fissure (space between the lesser and greater wings of the sphenoid, Fig. 2.7). Thus it gains access to the orbit where it divides to innervate levator palpebrae superioris, inferior oblique, and the superior, inferior and medial recti (see page 63). Within the brain stem there is a relay whereby a few visual axons from the optic radiation passing to the superior colliculus are able to stimulate parasympathetic nerve cells. Axons from these preganglionic fibres join the oculomotor nerve to pass to the orbit where they terminate in the small **ciliary ganglion** lying posteriorly in the orbit. From here the postganglionic parasympathetic nerve fibres, the **short ciliary nerves**, pass through the orbit to reach the globe and hence innervate the constrictor of the pupil, sphincter pupillae of the iris, and the ciliary muscle. The result of this reflex is such that shining a bright light into the eye results in constriction of the pupil.

Sweeping around the aqueduct from its nuclei is the **trochlear (fourth cranial) nerve**, which crosses the midline before leaving from the posterior surface of the midbrain in the posterior cranial fossa (Figs. 2.39, 2.44, 2.47). This very thin trochlear nerve passes laterally and anteriorly descending to cross the free edge of the tentorium cerebelli (from superior to inferior) before piercing the dura on the posterior aspect of the lateral wall of the cavernous sinus. Within the

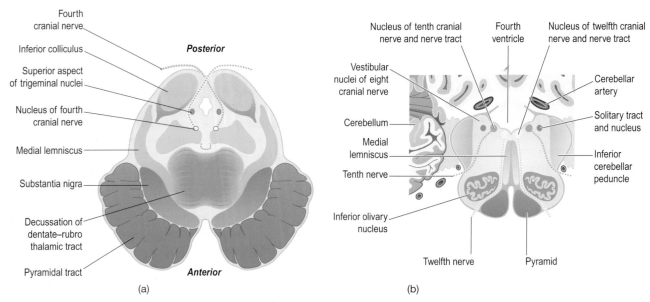

(a)   (b)

Fig. 2.47 Cross-sections of the hindbrain demonstrating key features of (a) midbrain, (b) medulla.

cavernous sinus it continues anteriorly to the superior orbital fissure to pass medially within the orbit to innervate the superior oblique muscle. With its long course within the CSF between the origin from the midbrain and where it pierces the dura, it is prone to damage, in particular from space-occupying lesions of the cerebral hemispheres, pushing the tentorium downwards. This movement can stretch this delicate nerve with a resultant paralysis of a single eye muscle, presenting clinically as double vision when a patient tries to turn the affected eye down and out.

The **trigeminal (fifth cranial) nerve** (Fig. 2.39) has a very extensive nucleus located superiorly in the midbrain and as far inferiorly as the distal medulla oblongata. This long nucleus passing through several regions of the brain stem reflects the mixed nature of the nerve, being sensory to the head and motor to the muscles of mastication. It leaves the surface of the brain on the anterolateral aspect of the pons (**cerebellopontine angle**) to pass over the superior aspect of the petrous part of the temporal bone to lie within a pocket of dura on the floor of the middle cranial fossa. Here this largely sensory nerve forms its main ganglia, the **trigeminal ganglion** (Fig. 2.37), from where its three main branches pass anteriorly and inferiorly to facial structures:

- The **first division (ophthalmic branch)** passes into the lateral wall of the cavernous sinus to reach the **superior orbital fissure** gaining access to the orbit. Thus it is in a position to be sensory to the forehead, anterior scalp, upper eyelid and the superior aspect of the nose. Its **nasociliary branch** passes medially in the orbit and gives general sensory branches to the ethmoidal air cells and the nasal mucosa in the superior aspect of the nasal septum and cavity.
- The **second division (maxillary branch)** passes in the floor of the cavernous sinus to reach the **foramen rotundum** in the floor of the middle cranial fossa. Passing through the pterygomaxillary fossa (space between the maxilla anteriorly and the pterygoid plates of the sphenoid posteriorly), the nerve passes into the maxilla to innervate the face between the upper lip, the lower eyelid and the lateral aspect of the orbit. In addition it provides the sensory supply to the nasal mucosa and the maxillary air sinus. It also provides innervation to the teeth of the upper jaw and, as such, it is not unknown for a patient to present with pain in the teeth of the upper jaw when they actually have an infection or tumour in the maxillary sinus.
- The **third division (mandibular nerve)** is a mixed nerve containing both sensory and motor nerve fibres. It descends by passing inferiorly from the trigeminal ganglion through the **foramen ovale** to lie just medial to the condyle of the mandible (Fig. 2.5). Its first branch passes horizontally and laterally between the base of the skull and lateral pterygoid muscle to reach the skin and temporalis on the lateral aspect of the skull. The remain-

ing branches, the **lingual** and **inferior alveolar**, descend to the mandibular foramen. Here the inferior alveolar branch passes into the mandible to innervate the teeth of the lower jaw, whilst the lingual nerve passes into the floor of the mouth. The sensory branches within the mandibular nerve innervate (a) skin over the mandible and just anterior to the ear, (b) the lower lip, (c) mucosa around the mandible within the oral cavity and (d) teeth of the lower jaw. The motor nerve fibres do not relay in the trigeminal ganglion but pass straight through to innervate (a) the muscles of mastication (temporalis, lateral and medial pterygoids, masseter and anterior belly of digastric), (b) mylohyoid, (c) tensor tympani and (d) tensor veli palatini.

Clinically the herpes zoster virus can infect one of the main sensory roots of the trigeminal nerve, with a resultant pain and rash in the distribution area of a single sensory root.

On the anterior aspect of the hindbrain between the pons superiorly and the medulla oblongata inferiorly, the small **abducent (sixth cranial) nerve** leaves the brain having passed anteriorly from its small nuclei located close to the floor of the fourth ventricle. It passes anteriorly to pierce the dura and ascend between the dura and the petrous part of the temporal bone to pass anteriorly in the floor of the cavernous sinus to pass through the superior orbital fissure to innervate the lateral rectus eye muscle.

A 45-year-old woman woke up with mild discomfort on the right side of her face. She also felt saliva dripping from the right corner of her mouth. When she looked in the mirror she was surprised to see that the lines on the right side of her face had gone and when she tried to smile or speak she noticed that her face twisted to the left. When she tried to drink her tea the fluid dribbled out of the right corner of her mouth. She went to see her family doctor who confirmed that the entire right side of her face was paralysed. In addition he noted she could not close her right eye and a tear trickled down her right cheek, her wrinkles on her forehead had gone and she could not lift her right eyebrow. When she tried to smile her smile was crooked.

Because the facial muscles were all affected on the right side above and below the eye, her GP told her that she had a Bell's palsy. The nerve involved was affected by a virus, after it had left the brain, and this was a lower motor neurone palsy. The doctor reassured her that this should get better in time. He prescribed some eye drops to protect the cornea from drying out until recovery occurred. He also prescribed a course of steroids to decrease the nerve swelling. Very gradually her facial nerve palsy improved but it took 3 months before recovery was complete. Even years later, after she had recovered, when she was tired, her friends noticed there was still some asymmetry of the right corner of her mouth.

ASSESSMENT *(cont'd)*

5. If patients aspirate, into which lung does the fluid or foreign body tend to pass and why?

She was referred to hospital. A barium swallow was performed (Fig. 2.53). This showed that she had developed a pouch on the left side of her neck arising from the pharynx.

6. Describe the anatomy of the pharynx as relating to the formation of a pouch.

7. Why did the old lady regurgitate foul-smelling food into her mouth?

8. Why did she have a persistent cough and repeated chest infections?

After the anatomy and pathology was explained to her she was offered an operation with one of the ENT specialists. Using a modern stapling device, the pouch was closed with a 'gun'. After this her chest gradually improved and she had no further episodes. She did well in the long term.

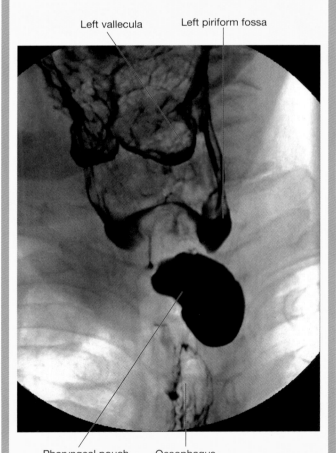

Left vallecula   Left piriform fossa

Pharyngeal pouch   Oesophagus

Fig. 2.53 Barium swallow demonstrating a pharyngeal pouch.

Case 3

A 70-year-old man who was a lifetime smoker had been keeping quite well until he suddenly developed, with no warning, weakness of his right arm and right leg. This lasted 12 hours and then improved spontaneously. He was referred to his family doctor for investigations. On examination in hospital, after 24 hours, the weakness had gone completely and he was back to normal health. His physicians thought he may have a 'transient ischaemic attack', caused by temporary blockage to the flow of blood in the middle cerebral artery.

9. Describe the blood supply to the cerebral hemispheres.

The physician, when she listened to his neck over the origin of the common carotid artery, heard a bruit (noise) of blood flow through a narrowed blood vessel on the left side.

10. At what level in the neck would one expect to hear a bruit?

11. Why did the patient then have symptoms on the right side of his body?

The Radiology Department was asked to perform a Doppler ultrasound scan. This revealed more than 70% narrowing of the origin of the internal carotid artery. A carotid arteriogram (Fig. 2.54a) confirmed this narrowing.

12. Why did the patient develop signs of a mini stroke?

13. What part of the brain is supplied by the middle cerebral artery?

The debris dispersed and the blood flow was restored. Because the origin of the internal carotid artery was narrowed, his physician was concerned that this could recur. She recommended surgery.

14. Describe the main relations of the bifurcation of the common carotid artery.

At operation the common carotid artery was exposed in the neck by an incision along the anterior border of sternomastoid. The surgeon found the common carotid artery within the carotid sheath, which also contains the internal jugular vein lying on the lateral aspect. The surgeon, having identified the blood vessels, found that the internal carotid artery was lateral to the external carotid artery and then passed medially and posteriorly to ascend along the pharynx with the internal jugular vein and the adjacent vagus nerve. The hypoglossal nerve lies in a curve superficial to the internal and external vessels.

15. How could the surgeon identify which vessel was the internal and which the external carotid artery?

ASSESSMENT (cont'd)

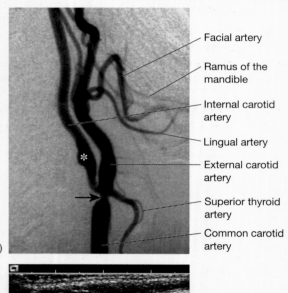

- Facial artery
- Ramus of the mandible
- Internal carotid artery
- Lingual artery
- External carotid artery
- Superior thyroid artery
- Common carotid artery

(a)

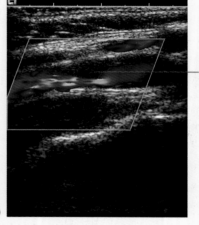

- Plaque narrowing artery

(b)

Fig. 2.54 (a) Selective left carotid arteriogram demonstrating carotid artery stenosis at the level of the bifurcation. Note the stenosis (→) in the common carotid and the posteriorly placed ulcer (*) on the internal carotid artery. (b) Doppler demonstrating narrowing at the level of the bifurcation.

Having clearly identified the major arteries, the surgeon occluded the common carotid and its two major branches (external and internal) and opened the blood vessels. He removed a plaque of atheroma, which had formed at the bifurcation of the common carotid artery. This operation is called an endarterectomy. The blood vessels were then closed and blood supply was restored to the brain. The most feared complication is death or a major stroke during the time of the occlusion of the internal carotid artery. The latter is dependent to some extent on the patency of the circle of Willis. Immediately after the patient had recovered from the anaesthesia, the patient was asked to move his limbs, particularly on the contralateral side. Movement can be monitored during surgery if the operation is performed under local anaesthesia. Following the operation the patient

made a satisfactory recovery. He was placed on Aspirin to prevent any further small clots forming and he had no further attacks.

Case 4

An 18-year-old girl went to her family doctor because she was concerned at having noticed a soft swelling on the right side of her neck. It was painless and had gradually increased in size over the previous few months. She had no other symptoms. On examination the family doctor noticed a soft swelling in the lateral aspect of her neck peeping around the corner of the right sternomastoid at the junction of the upper and middle one-third.

16. **Describe the anatomy and the nerve supply of the sternocleidomastoid muscle and its immediate relations.**

She was sent to hospital for investigations. An MR scan was performed and this showed a cyst containing fluid (Fig. 2.55). Because she was concerned about her appearance she wished to have the cyst removed. At surgery a soft cyst was found lying partially anteriorally and partially behind the sternomastoid muscle and containing dirty material including cholesterol crystals.

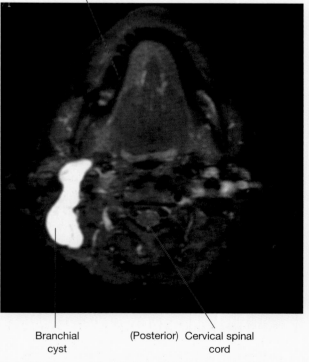

Teeth in mandible (Anterior)

Branchial cyst   (Posterior) Cervical spinal cord

Fig. 2.55 MR image of a right branchial cyst.

ASSESSMENT (cont'd)

The surgeon knew that this was a remnant of the second branchial arch. The surgeon removed the cyst and found there was a deep connection, which passed through the bifurcation of the common carotid artery between the internal and external carotid arteries. The connection extended towards the tonsil bed.

17. Describe the embryology of the branchial cyst (which explains the connection with the tonsil bed).

This was removed and the patient made a satisfactory and uneventful recovery.

Case 5

A 70-year-old man was referred by his family doctor because he had persistent hoarseness for 6 weeks. The family doctor knew he was a heavy smoker and he was concerned he had a tumour in his pharynx or larynx. The surgeon palpated the man's neck and found enlarged lymph nodes on the left side.

18. Describe the lymph drainage of the larynx.

His examination confirmed that he had a tumour of his vocal cords extending into the supraglottic area and this explained his hoarseness.

19. Outline the anatomy of the supraglottic area

The patient underwent the major operation of laryngectomy and a neck dissection to remove the lymph glands in his neck.

20. Describe the anatomy of the lymph glands in the lateral aspect of the neck.

The patient required a permanent tracheostomy and also required postoperative radiotherapy.

21. Describe the anatomy of the trachea and the immediate relations, which might be encountered by the surgeon performing a tracheostomy.

ANSWERS

1. *The symptoms suggest a possible tumour in his parotid gland that was pressing on the major divisions and branches of the facial nerve. The weakness of the upper division of the facial nerve caused flattening of his forehead and difficulty in closing his eye (temporal and zygomatic branches) and the weakness of the corner of his mouth was caused by pressure on the mandibular branch of the facial nerve. The other two branches (buccal and cervical) were less affected. Because the cervical branch supplies the platysma muscle it is difficult to detect damage to this particular nerve.*

2. *A needle biopsy would confirm a diagnosis and type of tumour of the left parotid gland, while an MRI scan (Fig. 2.56) would confirm the extent of the tumour.*

3. *At operation the parotid gland would lie within fascia inside which there may be some enlarged lymph glands. The facial nerve would be exposed running through the substance of the parotid gland separating it into superficial and deep lobes. The facial nerve could be traced back to the stylomastoid foramen where it emerges inferior to the bony part of the external auditory meatus. The parotid duct would lie anteriorly.*

4. *The patient would have a total facial nerve paralysis on the left side with flattening of the wrinkles on his forehead, an inability to close his eye (therefore, a risk of corneal damage) and drooping at the corner of the left side of his mouth.*

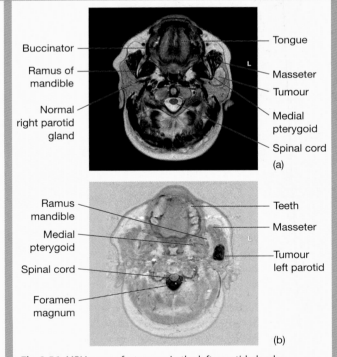

Buccinator — Tongue
Ramus of mandible — L
— Masseter
— Tumour
Normal right parotid gland — Medial pterygoid
— Spinal cord
(a)

Ramus mandible — Teeth
Medial pterygoid — Masseter
Spinal cord — Tumour left parotid
Foramen magnum
(b)

Fig. 2.56 MRI image of a tumour in the left parotid gland.

5. *Fluid and the foreign bodies tend to aspirate into the right lung because of the straighter, more vertical line of the right main bronchus.*

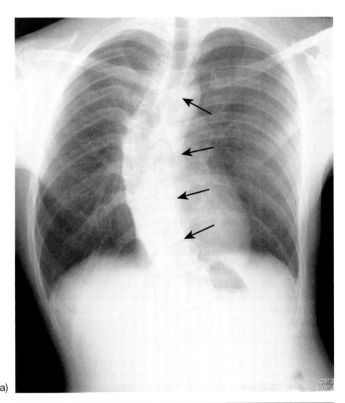

(a)

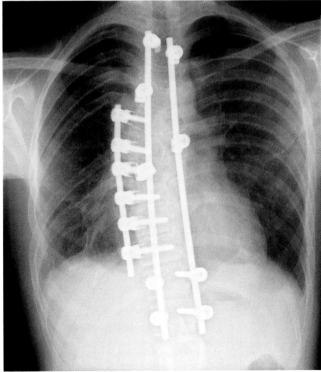

(b)

Fig. 3.10 Radiographs of a patient with scoliosis to the right (←): (a) preoperative and (b) postoperative, demonstrating the rods used to straighten the spine.

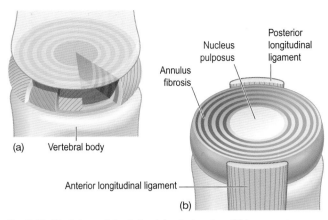

Fig. 3.11 The intervertebral disc: (a) anterior view, (b) transverse section.

Between adjacent vertebral bodies are the secondary cartilaginous joints known as intervertebral discs. Irrespective of their level they all have the same basic structure (Fig. 3.11). There is an outer ring of collagenous fibres, the **annulus fibrosus**, consisting of many layers of fibres which lie in different directions. Within the annulus is the softer (jelly-like) **nucleus pulposus**. Posteriorly the annulus is slightly thinner than anteriorly, and can rupture particularly in the lumbar region. Such a rupture allows the nucleus pulposus to herniate through the annulus and so press on structures leaving the vertebral canal through the intervertebral foramen, notably the spinal nerve at that level. In the lumbar region the discs become somewhat thicker anteriorly, especially between L4 and L5 and between L5 and S1 (Fig. 3.8).

A 52-year-old man presented to his general practitioner with longstanding back pain. Although this had been present for many years, it had worsened 2 weeks earlier after some gardening. Following this, the pain had become much worse and had radiated down his right leg. On examination, the patient was in obvious distress. Straight leg raising was reduced to 30° on the right, but was normal on the left. His general practitioner noted that his right ankle reflex was absent, although the left was normal.

His GP requested X-rays of the lumbar spine, which demonstrated a reduction of the disc space between L5 and S1, with osteophytes present at the margins of the vertebral bodies. At the recommendation of the radiologist a MRI scan was performed and it demonstrated a significant disc protrusion on the right side at the L5/S1 level (Fig. 3.12). This disc indented the thecal sac, and pressed against the right L5 and S1 nerve roots, thus explaining his pain and the loss of the ankle reflex. He was referred to a spinal surgeon.

The spinal surgeon discussed the pros and cons of surgery with the patient. He explained that 90% of disc protrusions settle conservatively. The patient's preference was for conservative management, and his symptoms settled with physiotherapy, weight loss and programmed exercise.

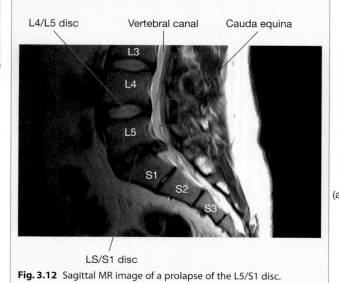

Fig. 3.12 Sagittal MR image of a prolapse of the L5/S1 disc.

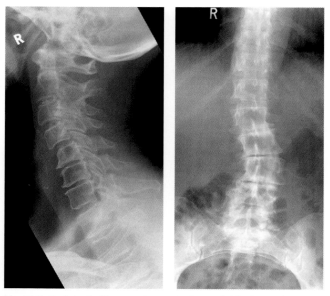

Fig. 3.13 Radiological images demonstrating arthritic change in (a) lateral cervical spine and (b) AP lumbar spine. Note the narrowing of the intervertebral discs and the lipping of the vertebral bodies.

Synovial joints

Posteriorly the articular facets form synovial joints. As with all synovial joints, the capsule passes from articular margin to articular margin, lined on non-articular surfaces by synovial membrane. Ligamentary support is from the larger ligaments detailed below. Within the capsule, particularly noticeable in the lumbar region, are small fat pads that project between the articular surfaces where the two articular surfaces are not always in contact. It has been postulated that sudden twisting movement could result in entrapment of these fatty pads, resulting in the presentation of an acute painful back. Being synovial joints they are prone to arthritic changes due to both osteoarthritis and rheumatoid arthritis (Fig. 3.13).

Ligaments

There are two longitudinal ligaments joining together all vertebral bodies, anteriorly the **anterior longitudinal ligament** and posteriorly the **posterior longitudinal ligament**. Both longitudinal ligaments are anchored superiorly to the occiput, the former through the **atlanto-occipital ligament** and the latter by the **membrana tectoria**. Inferiorly they attach to the sacrum. These important inelastic collagenous ligaments expand to attach to the superior and inferior edges of each vertebral body and the intervertebral disc between. Each ligament narrows as it crosses the waist of each vertebral body (Fig. 3.14). In some patients it is not unknown to find that the posterior longitudinal ligament has calcified in the cervical region, hence reducing neck mobility.

Joining adjacent lamina is an elastic ligament, the **ligamentum flavum** (Fig. 3.15). Elasticity here facilitates flexion of the spine whilst maintaining a smooth surface for the posterior aspect of the vertebral canal.

In the cervical spine an elastic ligament, the **ligamentum nuchae**, joins the tips of the spinous processes and the occiput. This has the function of limiting the range of flexion of one vertebra to the next, but being elastic provides a greater range of movement, as noted clinically, than would be possible if it was inelastic in nature.

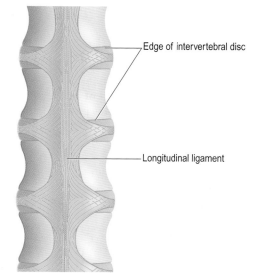

Fig. 3.14 A segment of the posterior longitudinal ligament.

LEARNING OUTCOMES

The reader should be able to:

❶ Identify and describe the main features of the typical cervical, thoracic and lumbar vertebrae and identify them on radiological images.

❷ Describe the first and second cervical vertebrae and identify them on radiological images.

❸ Describe the vertebral canal and intervertebral foramen and the relationship between these bony structures to the spinal cord and spinal nerves.

❹ Discuss the movement seen between adjacent vertebrae, the atlas and the skull, fifth lumbar vertebra and the sacrum.

❺ Discuss the structure and functional implications of the lumbar intervertebral disc.

❻ Describe the general pattern of the spinal musculature and how it controls spinal movement.

❼ Describe the normal curvature of the adult spinal column.

❽ Identify the vertebra prominens and vertebra level with the iliac crest.

❾ Describe the posterior articular facets and how their shape relates to function.

❿ Describe the blood supply and venous drainage of the spinal column.

⓫ Describe the lymphatic drainage of the spinal column.

⓬ Describe the gross anatomy of the spinal cord and the structure of a typical spinal nerve.

⓭ Describe the sympathetic outflow from the spinal cord.

⓮ Describe the form of the spinal cord and the spinal nerve roots at different levels and explain how this determines the choice of site for sampling cerebrospinal fluid (lumbar puncture) in the adult and child.

⓯ Describe the position and course of the major descending motor pathways within the central nervous system and determine the motor deficits that would result from lesions affecting different levels of the pathways.

⓰ Describe the position and course of the major ascending pathways within the central nervous system associated with pain, temperature and touch to understand the sensory deficits that would result from lesions affecting the sensory pathways.

ASSESSMENT

Case 1

A 37-year-old very fit man was playing rugby with his local club and during a line-out, while jumping, he was up-ended and came down on to his head and his neck became acutely flexed. He immediately lay still on the ground and as his colleagues approached him he yelled, 'Don't touch me because I have tingling in my fingertips'. He was a doctor and he knew to advise his colleagues not to move his neck in any way.

1. Why may this second row forward have tingling in his fingertips?

He had nerve root compression affecting C7 and C8 nerve roots. The tingling increased and he felt unable to move either hand. Then he also began to develop tingling in his toes.

2. What part of the nervous system could be affected to give him tingling in both arms in the region of his fingers and then also in his toes?

Wisely, he was placed very carefully on a stretcher with a neck brace in position so that his neck was not moved in any direction. He was taken very carefully to hospital. At

hospital he underwent a cervical spine X-ray without flexing his neck. Cervical spine X-ray showed a fracture in the region of C6 and C7 (Fig. 3.26). An MRI scan was also performed which confirmed this diagnosis.

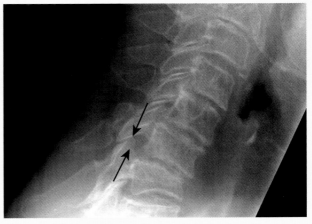

Fig. 3.26 Radiological image of the cervical spine: lateral demonstrating a subluxation of the C7 vertebral body (marked by →←).

ASSESSEMENT *(cont'd)*

3. Why was it so important not to flex his neck? How might neck movement make his injury worse?

With his head held rigidly in position he underwent careful spinal surgery to remove the bone fragments, which were impinging upon the anterior aspect of his spinal cord.

4. Describe the structures in the cord that could be compressed from these bone fragments pressing upon the cord from an anterior direction.

The spinal surgeon stabilised his spine with small plates and screws. Following surgery the numbness persisted in his fingertips for some months. The young man did not return to playing rugby!

Case 2

A 55-year-old man was moving house and he lifted a heavy table when he felt sudden pain in his lower back with immediate pain radiating down the lateral aspect of his right leg to his little toe. He collapsed on the ground, unable to move due to the severity of his pain. Despite pain relief and rest the pain became worse in his back. He had also noticed increasing numbness in the lower part of his foot on the lateral aspect.

5. What may have caused his acute back pain?

6. What may have caused his numbness in the lateral aspect of his foot?

His wife was gravely concerned and she called the ambulance and he was taken to the casualty department of his local hospital. He was noted to be in very severe pain. The examining doctor found that he had an absent ankle jerk and was unable to move his toes in an upward direction.

7. Describe the nerve damage that must have occurred to produce these signs.

An X-ray of the back was performed which showed an apparent narrowing of the disc space between L5 and S1. An MRI scan was performed which confirmed acute protrusion of his disc between L5 and S1 posteriorly. An orthopaedic surgeon specialising in back surgery was called. He further assessed the patient and found an area of numbness in his perineum around his anus.

8. Why was the patient numb around his anus?

The surgeon felt he needed urgent surgery but, while waiting for a theatre space, the patient found he was unable to pass urine and had to be catheterised.

9. Why could the patient not pass urine?

A theatre was rapidly made available and the surgeon performed a laminectomy through a posterior incision over his lower spine.

10. Describe the structures through which the surgeon would have to divide to get access to the prolapsed disc.

The traditional laminectomy is now being replaced with microdisectomy guided by highly accurate MR scanning.

Following his disc surgery the patient made a reasonable recovery, although the numbness in his little toe persisted for the rest of his life. Fortunately his bladder symptoms improved greatly although he still had some urinary symptoms and problems with erection.

11. Why might the patient have a problem with erection?

Case 3

A 25-year-old driver was admitted to the A&E department after his car had collided with a lorry. He had been wearing a seat-belt. He was conscious on admission, though in great pain, and complained specifically of breathlessness and left-sided chest and low back pain.

12. What could the chest X-ray show?

13. How would you treat fluid or air within the pleural cavity?

800 ml of blood was drained from the chest. Neurological examination of the lower limb was normal. The lumbar spine was X-rayed and then an urgent CT scan was requested (Fig. 3.27).

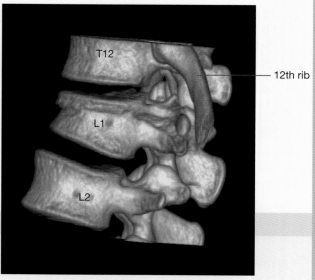

Fig. 3.27 CT reconstruction of the upper lumbar spine.

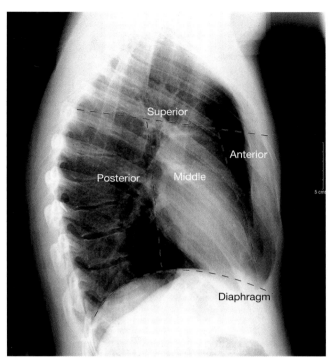

Fig. 4.13 Components of the mediastinum demonstrated on a lateral chest radiograph.

A 32-year-old man came to A&E with central chest pain that was worse on moving, especially when he lay down or took a deep breath. He had been complaining of flu-like symptoms the previous week. The doctor heard a pericardial rub (like a creaking shoe) when he listened to his heart and diagnosed pericarditis. Unfortunately the patient got worse the next day in hospital and became short of breath. The veins in his neck were distended. An echocardiogram showed a fluid collection around the heart within the pericardium – a pericardial effusion (Fig. 4.14). This tends to compress the heart as the parietal pericardium does not stretch and hence reduces the circulation of blood. The doctor had to drain this by passing

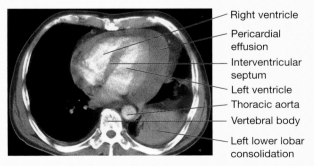

Right ventricle
Pericardial effusion
Interventricular septum
Left ventricle
Thoracic aorta
Vertebral body
Left lower lobar consolidation

Fig. 4.14 Axial CT image of the heart of a patient with a pericardial effusion.

a needle into the pericardium which improved the man's symptoms and he subsequently made a full recovery.

There are numerous causes of pericarditis but the most common are Coxsackie viral infections and after myocardial infarction.

Superior to the heart lie the main outflow vessels, the aorta and the pulmonary trunk, beside which on the right of midline lies the superior vena cava. The heart has an anterior, posterior, right, left and inferior surface (Figs. 4.15, 4.16). Within the heart there are four chambers, the two atria and two ventricles. The axis between the atria and ventricles runs obliquely from the right anteriorly, to the left posteriorly (Fig. 4.16), with the right atrium forming the right surface and the left atrium the posterior surface of the adult heart. The two ventricles form the anterior and most of the inferior (or diaphragmatic) surfaces while the left ventricle forms the left surface. Attached to each atrium is a blind pocket, the auricle or atrial appendage. There is a groove between the atria and ventricles within which lie the main stems of the coronary vessels that bring arterial blood to the heart muscle. From these stems branches pass to the various chambers passing down towards the apex of the ventricles. Unidirectional valves guard the direction of flow of blood within the heart to ensure that it normally passes from atrium to ventricle and ventricle to an artery. These are the cuspid valves (**tricuspid** and **mitral**) between atria and ventricle and the **semilunar** valves of the aorta and pulmonary trunk. All valves are anchored together to form the fibrous skeleton to which the myocardial cells attach (see below).

The right atrium (Fig. 4.15) superiorly receives blood from the head, neck and upper limbs through the **superior vena cava**, whilst inferiorly it receives blood from the abdomen, pelvis and lower limbs through the **inferior vena cava**. These three structures form the right edge of the mediastinum as seen on a chest X-ray (Fig. 4.1). On the anterior aspect lies a marked groove passing inferiorly from the base of the superior vena cava to the inferior vena cava, the **sulcus terminalis**, marking the boundary between the atria on the right and the auricle lying more on the antero-superior aspect of the atrium. The right auricle wraps medially around the right side of the aorta and pulmonary trunk.

On opening the right atrium with an incision between the superior and inferior vena cava, several features are obvious. Internally the sulcus terminalis is seen as a ridge, the **crista terminalis**. The internal surface of this chamber is smooth, though to the left of the crista terminalis, and passing into the auricle, the surface is ridged. These ridges, the **musculi pectinati**, represent the primitive atrial wall. Posteriorly on the smooth aspect of the internal surface is a shallow depression, the **fossa ovalis**, the remnant of the **foramen ovale** seen in fetal life (Fig. 4.17). Passing inferior to the fossa ovalis towards the opening of the inferior vena cava

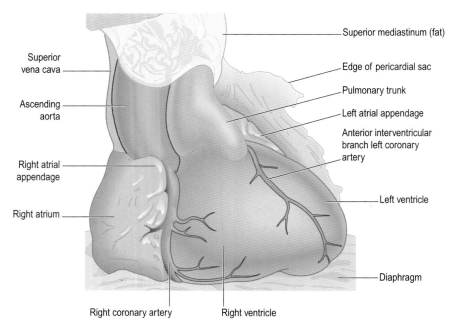

Fig. 4.15 Anterior view of the heart within the pericardial sac.

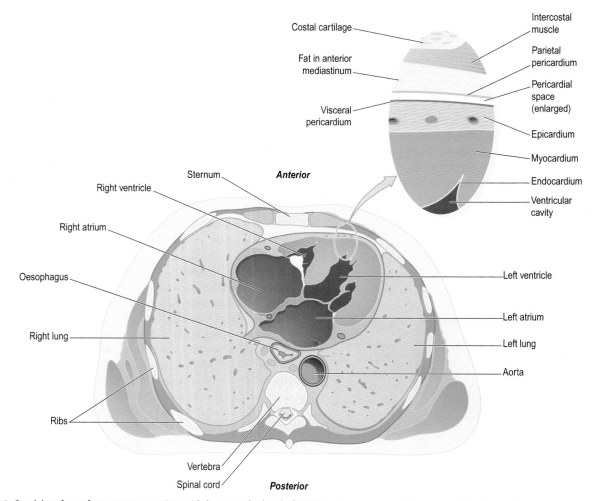

Fig. 4.16 Caudal surface of a transverse section mid-thorax at the level of T6/T7, with a close-up of the layers within the pericardial sac.

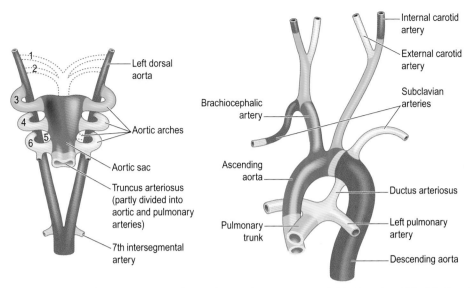

Fig. 4.32 The developing arterial arches (from Moore Persaud 1998 The Developing Human 6th Edn. Saunders, Philadelphia, with permission).

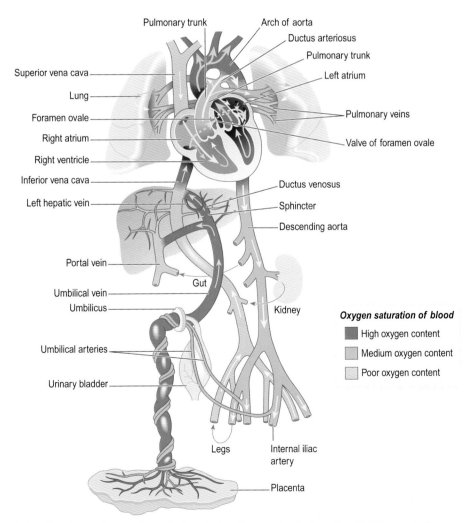

Fig. 4.33 The fetal circulation (from Moore Persaud 1998 The Developing Human 6th Edn. Saunders, Philadelphia, with permission).

adult circulatory pattern is established. Failure to close the truncus arteriosus results in a newborn baby that remains rather blue in colour as blood is able to bypass the lungs, hence the baby remains poorly oxygenated. Such children are taken to theatre early in life and the surgeon ties the truncus arteriosus, thus closing it. Instantly the child becomes pink as the blood is properly oxygenated.

RESPIRATORY SYSTEM

Pleural cavities

The right and left pleural cavities are lined with a serosal membrane, the pleura. As with other serosal lined cavities there is a parietal layer attached to the chest wall which continues inferiorly on to the superior surface of the diaphragm (diaphragmatic pleura) before continuing superiorly on the appropriate side of the mediastinum (mediastinal pleura). When the pleura reaches the hilum of the lung, it becomes continuous with the visceral pleura covering the surface of the lung. The pleural cavity is normally a closed space. Should this become open to the air, it becomes impossible to develop the necessary negative pressure to draw air into the alveolar spaces within the substance of the lungs. There are deep recesses between the parietal pleura inferiorly and the edges of the diaphragm, the **costodiaphragmatic recess** (Figs. 4.1, 4.2). Problems arise when the integrity of the pleural cavity is compromised.

John is a 22-year-old man who is very tall and thin. While studying at university one evening, he developed sudden pain in his chest and had great difficulty in breathing. He was taken urgently to hospital where the doctor examined him. When she listened to both sides of his chest she could detect no air entry on the left side. John was in a distressed state with increasing shortness of breath and was becoming a blue colour (cyanotic) because of insufficient oxygen getting into his blood. A chest X-ray was performed (Fig. 4.34) which revealed total collapse of the left lung. The left pleural space, which normally contains only a few millilitres of serous fluid, contained a massive amount of air. The doctor diagnosed that the patient had ruptured part of the lung and the air had leaked into the pleural space. She inserted a needle into the fifth intercostal space in the mid-axillary line. There was a whoosh as air immediately came out. John's condition improved dramatically. The shortness of breath improved and his colour returned to normal almost immediately.

A chest drain was inserted into the pleural space to remove any further air and this tube was inserted into a bottle (an underwater seal). Over the next 48 hours John's lung reinflated. There was no history of trauma and John's lung had collapsed because he had a cyst (bulla) in the upper portion of his left lung. This had burst spontaneously allowing the air inside the lung to enter the pleural space, causing collapse of that lung as more and more air was sucked out of the lung into the pleural space (because of the negative pressure in the pleural cavity). John made a full recovery, although he lost confidence for a while having found the experience very alarming and was frightened in case of recurrence.

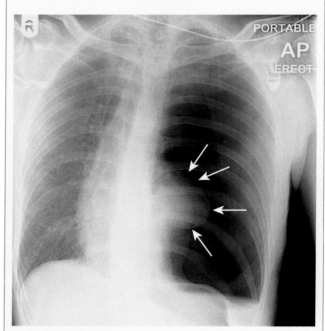

Fig. 4.34 Chest radiograph (PA) demonstrating a tension pneumothorax with a mediastinal shift to the right (← marks the edge of the left lung).

Access to the pleural cavity is required to drain fluid or air or to provide access to the organs within the chest. In both cases the same principles apply when passing through the intercostal space: the incision with a scalpel to cut the skin, followed by blunt dissection through the intercostal muscles or with a trochar, usually just superior to the upper border of a rib to avoid the neurovascular bundle (Fig. 4.10). The site is never just lateral to the sternum due to the presence of the internal thoracic artery and vein, nor is it within the first intercostal space. Care is taken if the lower intercostal spaces are used due to the domed nature of the diaphragm, as there is the risk of passing through the pleural cavity and piercing the abdominal cavity through the diaphragm; or on the right the liver is at risk.

The lungs

Each lung is joined to the mediastinal structures at the hilum where the main pulmonary veins and arteries pass to and from the heart. In addition there is the main airway. The structures at the hilum are ordered so that the pulmonary artery lies anterior and superiorly, with the pulmonary veins lying anterior and inferiorly. Posterior to the artery and superior to the pulmonary veins lies the main primary bronchus (Fig. 4.35). (N.B. The arrangement of these structures on dissected specimens varies considerably depending on whether the lungs were separated from the mediastinum, closer to the mediastinum or closer to the lung tissue.)

Macroscopically each lung is normally divided into three lobes on the right and two on the left (Fig. 4.36), each lobe supplied by a second-order bronchus (Fig. 4.37). Each

lobe is further subdivided as the hilar structures divide into **bronchopulmonary segments** and ultimately on to the alveolus. Names have been given to the bronchopulmonary segments as they are readily identified on a bronchogram, where each is supplied by a third-order bronchus. These segments are defined as functionally independent segments of lung supplied by a single branch of the pulmonary artery, vein and third-order bronchus.

The macroscopic shape of each lung is a result of the position of the heart which normally lies to the left of midline during development. This reduces the size of the medially positioned bronchopulmonary segments in the developing left lung to accommodate the heart. Located around the vessels at the hilum are the hilar lymph nodes, draining lymph from the lung tissue. In many individuals (especially city dwellers) these nodes are pigmented with the black carbon inhaled with respiration. The lung tissue when sectioned looks like a sponge and in life is very light and soft, being full of air. Superiorly the apex of the lung is level with or just above the first rib anteriorly whilst the inferior aspect (base) sits on the diaphragm.

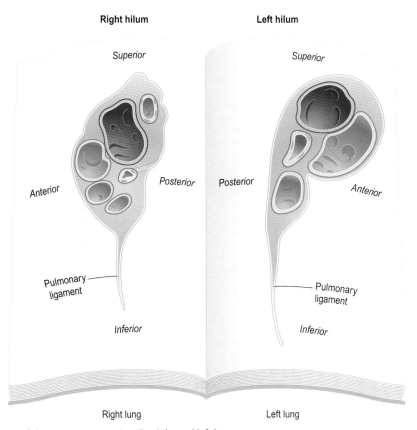

Fig. 4.35 The mediastinal view of the structures entering the right and left lungs.

ASSESSMENT *(cont'd)*

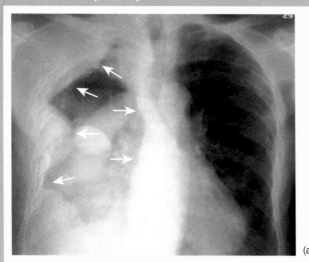

(a)

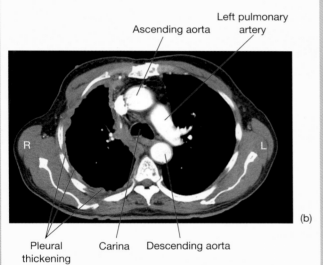

(b)

Pleural thickening   Carina   Descending aorta

Fig. 4.47 (a) PA chest radiograph demonstrating a right-sided mesothelial tumour and (b) CT scan of a right-sided mesothelioma (note the irregularity to the outline of the right pleural cavity compared to the left).

not operable. The patient was given chemotherapy and radiotherapy, but unfortunately he had little response and he passed away 6 months later.

Case 3

A 45-year-old man was driving his car when he was involved in a road traffic accident. He was not wearing his seat-belt. He was flung forward against the steering wheel. He developed immediate pain in his left chest and shortly afterwards became short of breath. He then felt increasingly faint, cold and sweaty. When the ambulance arrived, he was taken to hospital and was found to be in shock with a fast pulse rate and a low blood pressure. He

was extremely tender and bruised over his 6th and 7th ribs on the left side.

5. Which structures are likely to be damaged?

When the doctor listened to his chest he could hear no breath sounds in his left chest cavity. The patient was becoming increasingly short of breath.

6. Why no breath sounds on the left side of the chest?

A chest X-ray showed that he had fluid in his left pleural cavity filling almost the entire left side of his thorax. This fluid was compressing his lung and causing his shortness of breath. The trauma doctor inserted a chest drain into the pleural space on the left side. He inserted the drain immediately above the superior border of the 6th rib in the mid-axillary line. He inserted the drain in this position to avoid damaging the intercostal neurovascular bundle, which lies tucked in beneath the inferior border of the rib. Immediately 1 litre of blood came out through the drain and the patient's condition improved.

7. What vessel was most likely damaged in this case to produce so much bleeding?

The bleeding settled spontaneously with a blood transfusion and the patient improved. He was, however, very painful from his fractured ribs. He required an injection by the Anaesthetic Department to block the intercostal nerves. This led to great improvement in his pain relief and permitted physiotherapy, which allowed him to improve rapidly. In due course he made a full recovery.

Case 4

A 78-year-old woman complained to her GP of dizziness and frequent blackouts over a previous 4-week period. She had previously been well. The GP examined the patient and found a slow heart rate of 35 beats per minute but no other abnormality was noted. She was sent by her GP for a cardiograph. This showed the appearance of a complete heart block. This was caused by an interruption in the conduction system of the heart.

8. Describe the conduction system of the heart.

In elderly people the conduction is blocked at the level of the distal Purkinje fibres and the blackouts are called Stokes–Adams attacks. The patient was referred to hospital for insertion of a pacemaker.

9. Describe the venous route for insertion of the wires of a pacemaker to reach the appropriate part of the heart.

Following insertion of a pacemaker the problem with conduction was corrected and she made a full recovery.

ASSESSMENT *(cont'd)*

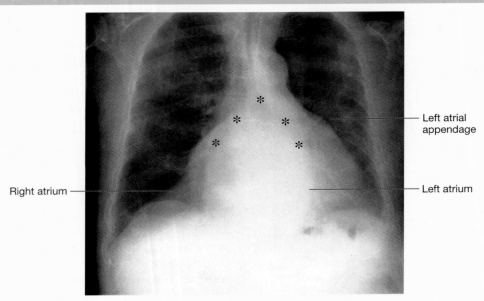

Fig. 4.48 Chest radiograph of mitral stenosis (** marks the outline of the left atrium).

Case 5

A 65-year-old woman had undergone a total hip replacement for very bad osteoarthritis 10 days ago. Her mobilisation after surgery was delayed by a chest infection (lobar pneumonia).

10. Describe the anatomy of the lobes of the lung.

Suddenly on the 10th postoperative day she felt sudden pain in her chest and extreme shortness of breath. The nurses noticed her to be collapsed and when she was examined it was noted that her pulse was racing and her blood pressure was low. Doctors were called and they were concerned that she had a clot in her legs (common after hip replacement). The clot (deep venous thrombosis) had moved in the circulation to lodge in her pulmonary artery (embolism).

11. Describe the anatomy of the pulmonary artery.

Her pulse was noticed to be very fast, her blood pressure was low.

12. Why did she have these cardiovascular changes?

The oxygen level in her blood fell and she appeared blue (cyanotic). It was also noted that the veins in her neck were distended.

13. Why were her neck veins distended?

A chest X-ray and CT were performed and demonstrated a thrombus in the pulmonary artery. A cardiograph showed some signs of right heart strain. An angiogram was carried

out. She was given oxygen and streptokinase was inserted in the pulmonary artery via a catheter to dissolve the clot in her pulmonary artery. She remained very ill for 48 hours and then gradually improved. She was then placed on Warfarin to keep her blood thin for life.

Case 6

A 68-year-old woman complained of fatigue, weakness and swelling of the legs. She had a past history of rheumatic fever as a child and she had been told previously that she had a heart murmur. She was examined by her doctor who heard a loud first heart sound followed by an opening snap as the mitral valve opens and early diastole with a rumbling, diastolic murmur at the apex of the heart.

14. Describe the anatomy of the mitral valve.

There were fine creps at the base of both lungs in keeping with mild pulmonary oedema (excess fluid in the lungs). A chest X-ray was performed.

15. Describe what might be expected in an X-ray of a patient with a narrowed (stenosed) mitral valve (Fig. 4.48).

An echocardiogram was performed and showed a narrowed mitral valve. She later required a mitral valve replacement and was prescribed Warfarin for life postoperatively. Mitral stenosis is commonly associated with rheumatic fever in the patient's youth and may take many years to reach a stage where it produces symptoms.

its opposite adduction across the trunk; medial and lateral rotation; and finally a combination of these movements, circumduction. (Clinically the anterior movement at the shoulder joint may be referred to as elevation.)

To deepen the glenoid fossa of the scapula there is a rim of fibrocartilage to increase the articular surface for the head of the humerus. However, there is an imperfect fit between the two, with the humeral articular surface being much larger than that of the glenoid. The capsule attaches from the articular margin of the glenoid to the articular margin of the humerus, except inferiorly where the capsule is reflected on to the surgical neck. Synovium lines the non-articular surfaces within the capsule. Three **glenohumeral ligaments** thicken the capsule itself which is reinforced superiorly by the **coracohumeral ligament**. However, while these support the joint they are insufficient to prevent dislocation of the joint when the muscles crossing the joint have been paralysed. Such a situation arises in a patient with a flaccid paralysis of the upper limb. If they did not wear a sling to support the weight of the limb, the joint would dislocate or sublux due to the effects of gravity.

The long head of biceps passes in the **intertubercular groove** (Fig. 5.10) to enter the joint cavity, lying superiorly within the cavity as it passes to the **supraglenoid tubercle** as a true intracapsular structure. External to the joint capsule is the **coracoacromial ligament**, which lies superior to the capsule separated from it by the **subacromial (subdeltoid) bursa**. This ligament helps to prevent, with the acromion, upward displacement of the head of the humerus. A group of muscles, the rotator cuff (see below), provides the key support to this joint preventing distraction of the humerus from the glenoid. However, there is still a weakness in the support and this is inferiorly where there is no ligament or muscular support, and this provides the commonest route for shoulder dislocation.

When observing movement of the shoulder joint (Table 5.1) it is important to ensure that the scapula is fixed, otherwise it is possible to exaggerate the range of movement observed. This occurs when the humerus reaches the end of the range of glenohumeral movement. Normally the scapula will rotate as appropriate to enhance the range of movement by changing the direction the glenoid fossa faces. When abduction occurs to 90° at the glenohumeral joint, the range is increased by lateral rotation of the scapula using trapezius. Therefore in assessing the range of shoulder joint movement, care must be taken to restrict scapular motion. However, when assessing the range of movement at the shoulder it is important to remember the range will involve movement of the shoulder girdle as well as the glenohumeral joint.

The **elbow joint** consists of two joints: (a) the humeroulnar-radial joint allowing flexion (anterior movement) from the anatomical position up to 150° (extension moves the joint to its straight anatomical position) (Table 5.1); (b) the proximal **radioulnar** joint permitting **pronation** and **supination** (rotation of forearm around the ulna). In effect the two joint spaces are continuous (Fig. 5.11).

The capsule of the elbow joint passes from the articular margin of the humerus proximally to the articular margins of the radius and ulna distally. Being a hinge joint, the elbow joint has **two collateral ligaments**. On the medial side, the medial or ulnar collateral ligament fans out distally from the medial epicondyle (Fig. 5.11) to the medial surface of the olecranon and coronoid process. Laterally, the lateral or radial collateral ligament fans distally from the lateral epicondyle to the lateral aspect of the ulna directly and through blending with the annular ligament, which in turn is very firmly attached to the lateral aspect of the proximal ulna. The **annular ligament** is the key structure maintaining the

Table 5.1   RANGE OF MOVEMENT OF THE MAIN UPPER LIMB JOINTS

	SHOULDER (GLENOHUMERAL) JOINT	ELBOW (HUMEROULNAR) JOINT
Flexion	90°	150°
Extension	60°	0°
Abduction	90°	–
Adduction	50°	–
Medial (internal) rotation	90°	–
Lateral (external) rotation	60–80°	–

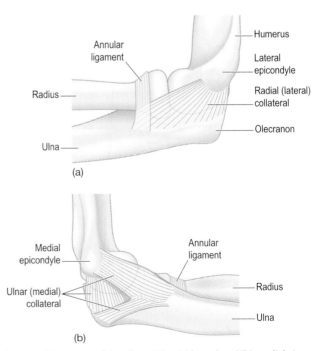

Fig. 5.11 Ligaments of the elbow joint: (a) lateral and (b) medial views.

proximal radioulnar joint by holding the radius firmly against the ulna. It attaches anteriorly and posteriorly to the lateral aspect of the ulna, running around the neck of the radius to form a tight sling around the narrow radial neck. The proximal synovial radioulnar joint has a capsule enclosing, and communicating with, the main capsule of the elbow joint, an arrangement ideally suited to maintain the radius against the ulna and humerus, allowing the radius to rotate around the fixed axis of the ulna.

The **distal radioulnar joint** has a weak capsule and is reinforced through the ligaments joining the radius and ulna to the carpal bones. This joint space is separated from the carpal bones by the ulnar disc, which joins the medial aspect of the radius and the ulnar styloid process. Working with the proximal radioulnar joint, both of these pivot joints facilitate the movements of pronation and supination. This rotational movement of the forearm allows the wrist and hand to be positioned in the optimal position for the function required. The interosseous membrane, a layer of thick fascia passing the full length of the forearm between the two radioulnar joints, further binds the shafts of the radius and ulna together.

At the wrist, the **intercarpal joints** are in effect two hinge joints placed at approximately 90° to each other. In one plane there is flexion (anterior movement of the hand from the anatomical position) and its opposite extension; in the other plane there is abduction (or radial deviation) movement laterally from the anatomical position and its opposite adduction (or ulnar deviation).

The distal radius articulates (Fig. 5.5) with the scaphoid laterally, the lunate more medially, and is attached to the same by short ligaments on both dorsal and palmar aspects. The distal ulna articulates through a fibrous disc with the triquetral bone and laterally the distal radius. When viewing the wrist as a whole there are three key joint spaces (Fig. 5.12): (1) proximally between the carpus and the distal radius (and ulna), (2) the intercarpus (between proximal and distal rows) and (3) distally between the carpus and the

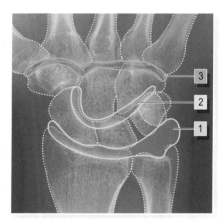

Fig. 5.12 The main joint spaces of the wrist joint: (1) proximal, (2) intermediate, (3) distal.

metacarpals. Laterally the joint space between the trapezium and the first metacarpal, a saddle-shaped joint, is also separate from the main intercarpal joint space. The carpal and metacarpal bones act as a unit pivoting with the radius around the distal ulna in pronation and supination of the forearm. This carries with it the first metacarpophalangeal joint. Between all bones are small ligaments joining adjacent osseous structures to maintain position and allow the minimal movement between each to support function.

The **metacarpophalangeal** and **interphalangeal** joints are basically hinge joints and as such all have medially and laterally placed **collateral ligaments**. In addition there is a ligament on the palmar aspect of each joint to limit the range of extension. The condylar nature of the metacarpal head allows for the slight abduction and adduction observed with the medial four fingers at the metacarpophalangeal joint. Abduction and adduction of the thumb occur at the carpo-metacarpal joint rather than at the metacarpophalangeal joint. Here the saddle-shaped joint allows for the full range of movement, flexion, extension, abduction, adduction and the rotational element required for opposition.

Muscles

A 40-year-old builder fell off a roof. As he fell, he reached out with his right hand and caught some scaffolding to stop himself falling further. He felt his right shoulder wrench and had a lot of pain around his shoulder. Unable to carry on at work, he went to A&E. On examination he had a decreased range of movement due to pain around his right shoulder with pain radiating down his arms. He was unable to abduct or externally rotate his arms and could not put his right hand behind his head.

X-rays were performed to make sure he had not dislocated the shoulder and these were normal. An ultrasound scan of his shoulder was performed and this demonstrated a full thickness tear of the supraspinatus tendon with fluid in the long head of the biceps tendon. He was treated surgically with an arthroscopic assessment of the tear and then a surgical repair of the tendons. He recovered very well and was able to return to work some months later.

The musculature can be divided in several different ways by function, by anatomical position or a combination of both. Muscles that lie anterior to the chest or anterior to a joint in the limb tend to flex the joint they cross. Likewise muscles on the posterior aspect of the chest or posterior to a joint tend to extend that joint. Providing the articular surfaces allow, muscles passing to the lateral aspect of a joint will abduct, whereas muscles on the medial side will tend to adduct.

It is useful to think of the muscles passing from the chest wall to the limb girdle as positioning muscles (Table 5.2). They position the scapula to enhance the range of positions

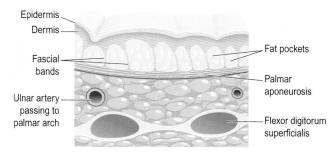

Fig. 5.19 Cross-section through the palmar skin.

In the palm of the hand the long digital flexor tendons lie between the thenar eminence (soft swelling on the palmar aspect) of the thumb laterally and the hypothenar eminence (the soft swelling of the palmar aspect of the 5th metacarpal) of the little finger medially. Flexor digitorum superficialis (Tables 5.5 and 5.6) lies superficial to flexor digitorum profundus tendon, splitting (Fig. 5.20) to pass either side of the profundus tendon before rejoining to pass and attach to the middle phalanx. This split forms a 'ring' around profundus just distal to the metacarpophalangeal (MCP) joint. Attaching to each of the profundus tendons is a lumbrical muscle whose role is vital to ensure a normal 'digital sweep' of the medial four digits. The small lumbrical muscles contract with profundus and through their attachments, passing anterior to the MCP joint and posterior to the interphalangeal (IP) joints, are able to ensure that the MCP joint flexes before the IP joints are able to flex. (Should one or more lumbrical muscles cease to function, the affected digit(s) will 'claw' with flexion of the interphalangeal joints before the metacarpophalangeal joint. This results in flexion of the distal inter-

phalangeal (DIP) joint first when digitorum profundus contracts, then the proximal interphalangeal (PIP) joint and finally the MCP joint flex.)

The expanded **extensor digitorum tendon** (Fig. 5.21) provides attachment for the **lumbrical** and **interossei** of the medial four digits. It provides the main extensor force for the medial four digits, extending the metacarpophalangeal and interphalangeal joints. The long flexor tendons are held in place against the phalanges by the flexor sheath, a tough fascial sleeve, which is thickened in the plane of each joint to form the digital pulleys. Each of the digits is also capable of abduction from, and adduction to, the middle finger. The **palmar interossei** are responsible for adduction of the little, ring and index fingers to the middle finger while the thumb is adducted by adductor pollicis. Apart from the little finger and thumb (which have their own dedicated abductors), the **dorsal interossei** abduct the index and middle fingers laterally and the middle and ring fingers medially.

Important in understanding movement of the thumb is its resting position, where the palmar aspect of the thumb lies at right angles to the plane of the palm of the hand (Fig. 5.22). Abduction moves the thumb at right angles to the palm, flexion and extension occur in the plane of the palm. It is the ability of the small muscles, especially the opponens pollicis and abductor pollicis, to 'rotate' the first MCP joint that makes us unique. Opposition allows the thumb to move into a position where it is able to oppose the other digits through pulp to pulp contact. This movement greatly enhances the functionality of the hand and is key to the majority of functions requested by modern lifestyle, being important in the **pinch grip**, used in writing and manipulating small objects. Without it we have the strong grasp type of grip seen so prominently in infants and the great apes.

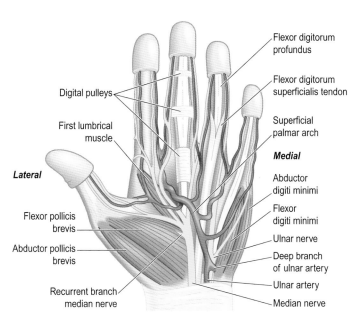

Fig. 5.20 Superficial muscles of the palm of the left hand.

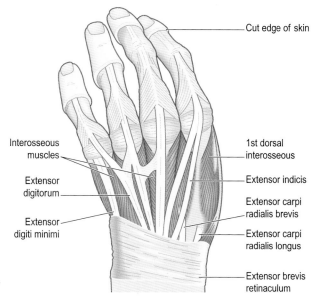

Fig. 5.21 Extensor tendons on the dorsum of the left hand.

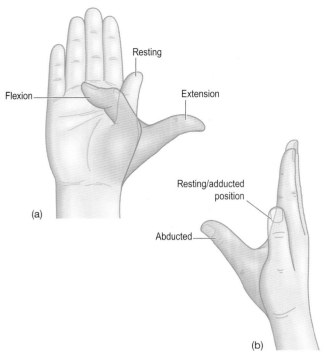

Fig. 5.22 Resting position and movement of the thumb: (a) palmar and (b) lateral views.

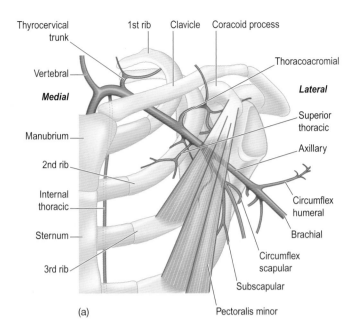

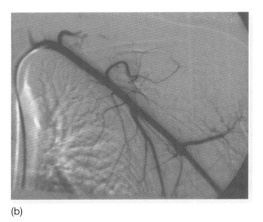

Fig. 5.23 Subclavian and axillary arteries of the left shoulder: (a) diagrammatic representation of the vessels demonstrated in the arteriogram (b).

CARDIOVASCULAR SYSTEM

Arterial supply

The **subclavian arteries** provide the main arterial supply to each upper limb. On the right it normally branches from the **brachiocephalic artery**, whilst on the left it is a direct branch of the arch of aorta. Passing laterally the subclavian artery lies superior to the upper surface of the first rib (Fig. 5.23), lying posterior to the scalene tubercle to which the neck muscle scalenus anterior attaches (see Chapter 3). Just proximal to the first rib there is the important branch, the **vertebral artery**, passing posteriorly to the foramen transversarium of C6 on each side, before it passes cranially. More anteriorly there are the smaller branches, (a) the **thyrocervical trunk**, supplying the thyroid gland via the inferior thyroid artery and the suprascapular and transverse cervical arteries passing to supply muscles of the shoulder, and (b) the **internal thoracic artery** (see page 108). As the subclavian artery crosses the lateral border of the first rib it becomes known as the **axillary artery**.

Proximally the **axillary artery** has several branches (Fig. 5.23), (1) anteriorly the **thoracoacromial artery**, passing along the pectoral muscles, and giving the superior and lateral thoracic arteries, (2) inferiorly lies the **large subscapular artery** and (3) passing posteriorly around the scapula, the **circumflex scapular artery**. Surrounding the scapula is an anastomotic network formed by the subscapular, circumflex scapular and the branches of the thyrocervical trunk. Finally, as the axillary artery descends into the arm it gives rise to the anterior and posterior **circumflex humeral arteries** passing round the surgical neck of humerus. In the axilla the axillary artery is surrounded by an extension of the prevertebral fascia, ensuring a close approximation of the cords and branches of the brachial plexus (see below) to the artery.

Distal to the lower border of teres major the axillary artery becomes the **brachial artery** (Fig. 5.24a), which descends on the medial aspect of the arm accompanied by the median nerve and brachial vein. Just proximal to the cubital fossa the neurovascular bundle comes more anteriorly to pass superficial to brachialis and lateral to the origin of the common flexor muscles attaching to the medial epicondyle. At this

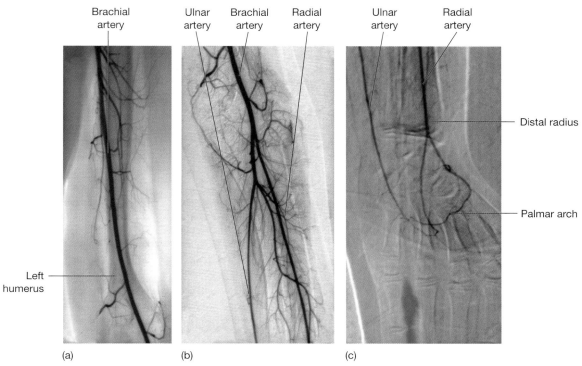

Fig. 5.24 Arteriogram of the left upper limb: (a) the arm, (b) cubital fossa and forearm, (c) the hand.

point the artery is easily palpated and auscultated when manually recording a patient's blood pressure. Normally the brachial artery and median nerve lie deep to the deep fascia and the bicipital aponeurosis. The brachial artery passes into the cubital fossa, where it normally divides into two terminal branches, the **ulnar** and **radial** arteries (Fig. 5.24b), which pass distally into the forearm. Medially the ulnar artery passes deep to pronator teres, deep to the other common flexor muscles to gain access to the deep surface of flexor carpi ulnaris. Here it continues distally and runs along the lateral side of the ulnar nerve passing to the wrist where it is palpable lateral to flexor carpi ulnaris and medial to flexor digitorum superficialis. It lies on flexor digitorum profundus throughout most of its course.

An 8-year-old boy presented to the A&E department following a 2 metre fall from his garden fence. He was complaining of severe pain and restricted movement of his right elbow. On examination, he was acutely tender over the elbow. The right radial pulse, although reduced, was present. He was not able to extend his own elbow beyond 70°. No attempt was made to actively extend the child's elbow, as the A&E physician suspected a supracondylar fracture of the right elbow.

Radiographs of the right elbow confirmed the clinical diagnosis of a displaced supracondylar fracture of the right humerus. The child was reviewed by the orthopaedic team and the decision was made to reduce the fracture in theatre and maintain the reduction with wires. Following reduction, the radial pulse became strong. There was no subsequent neurological defect in the median nerve distribution.

Passing anterior to the carpal bones (Figs. 5.24c, 5.25), the **ulnar artery** (lying lateral to the ulnar nerve and the pisiform bone) divides giving a **deep** and **superficial branch**. The latter passes laterally just deep to the palmar fascia to anastomose with the superficial branch of the radial artery to form the **superficial palmar** arch, level with the distal aspect of the metacarpophalangeal joint of the thumb. Passing through the hypothenar muscles the deep branch comes to lie deep to the tendons of flexor digitorum profundus to anastomose with the radial artery forming the **deep palmar arterial arch**. Both arches give rise to metacarpal arteries, which anastomose near the metacarpal heads to form **common palmar digital arteries**. On reaching the base of the cleft between adjacent fingers, the web space, they divide to give one branch to the sides of adjacent fingers. As a result each digit has a single digital artery on the medial and lateral sides. The ulnar artery normally provides the main arterial supply to the superficial palmar arch.

Laterally the **radial artery** lies more superficially, just deep to brachioradialis, passing distally to have a more exposed length (cf. ulnar artery) to lie lateral to flexor carpi radialis proximal to the wrist. It is this artery that is normally used

A 30-year-old man who was a passenger in a vehicle was involved in a road traffic accident. He was not wearing a seat-belt and was flung out of the vehicle. When he was taken to hospital his main symptoms were pain and swelling around the shaft of the left humerus. He also complained of an inability to extend his wrist on that side.

On examination the patient was found to have wrist drop due to paralysis of the muscles of extension and there was a small area of decreased sensation on the dorsum of the hand between the first and second metacarpals. The X-ray (Fig. 5.31) of the left upper arm showed that there was a fracture of the humerus at the midpoint of the shaft and this correlated with injury to the radial nerve.

The orthopaedic surgeon stabilised the fracture with a plate, then the plastic surgeon repaired the divided radial nerve. However, because this is a complex motor and sensory nerve, 6 months after the operation there was little recovery. The patient had to wear a splint and found great difficulty in gripping objects in his hand. Future surgery will be con-templated, either a nerve graft procedure, or if this failed, a tendon transfer to improve the wrist function. The small area of decreased sensation did not concern the patient.

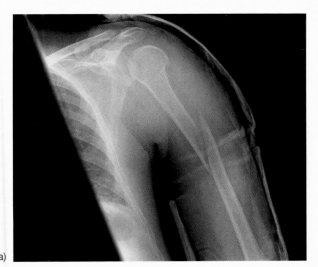
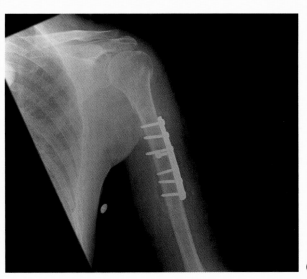

(a) (b)

Fig. 5.31 Fractured left humerus: (a) preoperative, (b) postoperative demonstrating a plate fixing the fracture site.

The **musculocutaneous nerve** normally pierces coraco-brachialis before passing distally in the anterior compart-ment of the arm, deep to biceps and superficial to brachialis. It innervates all of these muscles before emerging lateral to biceps tendon as the **lateral cutaneous nerve of the forearm**. This nerve contains nerve fibres from the C5, C6 and C7 roots of the plexus.

The **median nerve** passes distally with the brachial artery on the medial aspect of the forearm. It lies medial to biceps tendon before passing deep to the two heads of pronator teres, crossing the ulnar artery to lie deep to flexor digitorum superficialis. Here the median nerve supplies all muscles of the anterior forearm *except* flexor carpi ulnaris and the ulnar half of flexor digitorum profundus. In the distal forearm it passes laterally to emerge just proximal to the wrist lateral to the long superficial flexors. It then turns medially and anteriorly to lie superficial to the long flexor tendons as it passes into the carpal tunnel. Normally it gives its **recurrent branch** to the thenar muscles distal to this tunnel, but in a significant number of individuals this branch can arise either proximal to, or deep to, the flexor retinaculum. In the carpal tunnel space is limited and the median nerve is likely to be compressed if there is swelling of the connective tissue sur-rounding the digital tendons, giving rise to the **carpal tunnel syndrome**. In the hand it supplies skin of the palmar aspect of the lateral three and a half digits, muscles of the thenar eminence and lateral two lumbrical muscles. This nerve con-tains nerve fibres from all five roots of the plexus.

A 75-year-old woman visited her family doctor complaining of numbness in her right thumb, forefinger and middle finger with quite severe pain in those fingers, especially at night-time. She was also having difficulty in doing up her buttons, writing, and could no longer sew. When the doctor examined her, he found that she had decreased sensation over the palmar surface of thumb, forefinger and middle finger only; other areas of the hand were normal. He also noticed that there was very severe wasting and weakness of the muscles of the thenar eminence. Nerve conduction studies confirmed that the median nerve had decreased conduction at the level of the wrist, indicative of compression in the carpal tunnel.

The surgeon operated upon her wrist and found that the median nerve was significantly compressed. The flexor retinaculum was divided towards the ulnar side of the mid-point of the retinaculum, in a proximal/distal direction. This released pressure on the nerve. 24 hours after the operation the pain had gone from her hand, but it took 6 months after surgery for the muscle power of the thenar eminence to recover and the numbness to improve. However, because the severe night-time pain was gone the patient was satisfied with the results of her surgery.

The **ulnar nerve** passes slightly posterior to the brachial artery in the upper arm before passing through the intermuscular septum, to lie on the medial head of triceps. It then passes posterior to the medial epicondyle between the two heads of flexor carpi ulnaris to run deep to this muscle and superficial to the ulnar aspect of flexor digitorum profundus. As it reaches the wrist it passes, lateral to the pisiform bone and superficial to the flexor retinaculum, into the palm of the hand. Dividing into **superficial** and **deep branches** (Fig. 5.32), the deep branch accompanies the deep branch of the ulnar artery passing laterally towards the first metacarpal. The ulnar nerve supplies the two muscles in the forearm (which it lies between), the hypothenar and interosseous muscles, the medial two lumbrical muscles and adductor pollicis. In

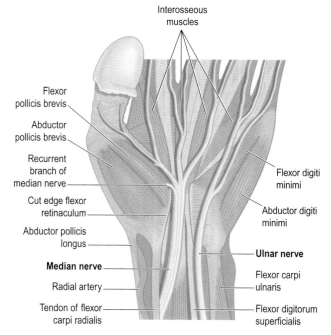

Interosseous muscles

Flexor pollicis brevis

Abductor pollicis brevis

Recurrent branch of median nerve

Cut edge flexor retinaculum

Abductor pollicis longus

Median nerve

Radial artery

Tendon of flexor carpi radialis

Flexor digiti minimi

Abductor digiti minimi

Ulnar nerve

Flexor carpi ulnaris

Flexor digitorum superficialis

Fig. 5.32 Nerves of the palm of the hand.

some individuals it also supplies flexor pollicis brevis and occasionally opponens pollicis. This nerve contains C8 and T1 nerve fibres from the plexus.

Each finger has four **digital nerves** supplying it, two on the palmar aspect, one on each side of the finger, and two on the dorsal aspect, again one each side, e.g. the index finger will have two palmar branches from the median nerve and two dorsal branches from the radial nerve. The digital artery lies on the dorsal side of the palmar digital nerve (Fig. 5.20).

There are several at-risk sites where a fracture of the underlying bone will compromise vital structures in the upper limb. These sites and clinical features are:

1. Surgical neck of humerus – **axillary nerve** – damage in shoulder dislocation or fractured neck of humerus – clinical sign: numbness in lateral aspect of arm distal to acromion.
2. Mid-shaft humerus – **radial nerve** – fracture – clinical sign: weakness in wrist extensors seen as a 'wrist drop'. Ask patient to extend wrist, with the palm of the hand at right angles to the table top to neutralise gravity, and test skin sensation on the dorsum of the hand over 1st and 2nd metacarpals.
3. Distal humerus – **brachial artery** – fracture in children, distal fragment projects anteriorly compressing the artery or causing an intimal tear – clinical sign: loss of radial pulse and/or ulnar pulse in presence of a fracture.
4. Medial epicondyle – **ulnar nerve** – fracture – clinical sign: weakness of the intrinsic muscles of the hand. Test the ability to abduct and adduct the fingers, also test for a loss of sensation over palm and dorsum of 5th metacarpal (the hypothenar eminence). There may also be a mild clawing of the hand.
5. Carpal tunnel – **median nerve** – compression due to long flexor tendon inflammation or arthritis – clinical signs: tingling in median distribution of the palm of the hand, weakness in pinch grip and tapping of a finger on the carpal tunnel will elicit discomfort in the area of median nerve distribution (Tinel's sign). Test ability to *maintain* (against resistance) pulp to pulp position of thumb and ring or middle finger and sensation over the palmar aspect of the index finger and the palmar area between the radial (lateral) two metacarpals. (N.B. It has been reported that the median and ulnar nerves may both innervate opponens pollicis. In such patients it has been suggested that the more appropriate test for the median nerve would be testing abductor pollicis brevis alone. Ask the patient to abduct the thumb and palpate the muscle at the same time to check that it is tense. However, caution is required to ensure that the action of abductor pollicis longus, radial nerve innervated, is not tested in error. Nerve problems can now be accurately identified by nerve conduction studies.)

layer that might occur. However, visceral peritoneum receives innervation from the autonomic nervous system and irritation of this layer is poorly localised, usually to the central region.

Embryology

It is easier to understand this cavity by thinking of the development of the abdominal portion of the gastrointestinal tract. The gut tube is formed by embryonic folding during the fourth week of intrauterine life, which brings the endodermal surfaces together. It comprises a blind-ended cranial **foregut**, a **midgut** open to the yolk sac and a blind-ended caudal **hindgut**. The lumen of this gut tube is filled by proliferating epithelial cells before it gradually recanalises. Hence in early fetal life the **coelomic (abdominal) cavity** contains a straight gut tube passing from the developing diaphragm to the primitive genital cleft. It is suspended from the posterior abdominal wall by three vessels passing from the aorta. The most cranial vessel supplies the abdominal **foregut**, the middle vessel supplies the **midgut** and the most caudal vessel supplies the **hindgut**. Developing serosal membrane covering the cavity wall is reflected from the posterior abdominal wall to pass on both sides of these vessels to meet on the surface of the gut tube to form the dorsal mesentery (Fig. 6.6a). Eventually this will form the **greater omentum** and mesenteries for the small intestine, transverse colon and sigmoid colon. The foregut region is also fixed to the anterior abdominal wall by another double fold of serosal membrane, the ventral mesentery. However, here the mesentery is also reflected off the diaphragm and surrounds the umbilical vein returning blood from the placenta via the umbilicus to pass through the diaphragm to the heart. In the adult this will become the **falciform ligament** and the **lesser omentum**. Also connected to the future anterior abdominal wall at the future umbilicus is the **vitellointestinal duct**, passing from the primitive yoke sac outside the body cavity to the midpoint of the midgut. The serosal covering of this structure, however, does not form a mesentery, as this connection is normally lost in fetal life.

The abdominal **fetal foregut** will form the abdominal **oesophagus**, **stomach** and the first two parts of the duodenum by the fifth week. The stomach walls produce the greater and lesser curvatures by differential growth and then, during the sixth and seventh weeks, the stomach rotates around its longitudinal axes so that the greater curvature is finally directed to the left and slightly caudally (Fig. 6.6). The rotation forms a space dorsal to the rotated stomach and dorsal mesogastrium, which will become the **lesser sac** of the peritoneal cavity. On the left lateral boundary of the stomach a pouch of dorsal mesogastrium is formed, which will give rise to the greater omentum that will lie superficial to and cover the abdominal viscera inferiorly.

At the same time within the ventral mesentery the liver and biliary system start to develop, dividing the mesentery

to leave a part between the gut tube and liver; this will form the **lesser omentum** with the biliary duct in its free edge. The developing liver will fall to the right where there is more space within the coelomic cavity, as the heart is usually developing and pressing down on the left. This fall of the liver pushes the foregut to the left assisting in creating a bulge in the dorsal mesentery, which will start to form the greater omentum (Fig. 6.6).

The **fetal midgut** differentiates into the remaining distal two parts of the duodenum, jejunum, ileum, caecum, ascending colon and proximal two-thirds of the transverse colon. The midgut starts to lengthen due to growth of the ileum resulting in an anteroposterior folding, the primary intestinal loop, on either side of the middle artery along the axis of the vitellointestinal duct towards the umbilicus. This occurs at the same time as the foregut develops a bulge in the fifth week. As the peritoneal cavity is too small, the midgut loop herniates through the umbilicus. During herniation, the bowel loop rotates around its long axis (of the vitellointestinal duct) by 90° in an anticlockwise direction, leaving the proximal (small bowel) component lying to the left and the large bowel component on the right. After the tenth week, the intestinal loop reduces back into the abdominal cavity and rotates through a further 180° in an anticlockwise direction producing the configuration of the small and large intestines.

The proximal component of the midgut will become more convoluted on the left side of the cavity to form the small intestine, whilst the distal component will become the terminal ileum, caecum, ascending and proximal two-thirds of the transverse colon, all supplied through a single branch of the aorta. Through the rotation of midgut and the movement of the liver, the joining parts of fore- and midgut (to become the duodenal loop) now come to lie posterior to the distal midgut loop. Progressively this interface area becomes less able to move and the mesentery is lost posteriorly, therefore the gut tube now makes contact with the posterior abdominal wall. Contact with the posterior abdominal wall by the ascending and descending large bowel results in the gradual resorption of the dorsal mesentery, resulting in the definitive structures becoming retroperitoneal. During this time the distal midgut will elongate towards the liver on the right before it descends on the right normally into the pelvic cavity. In doing so it drags the developing ileum and appendix with it. Once in the pelvis the caecum ascends to take up its normal adult position in the right iliac fossa (Fig. 6.6).

The **hindgut** forms the remaining part of the **transverse**, **descending** and **sigmoid colon** and the upper two-thirds of the **rectum**, and following rotation of the midgut the hindgut is pushed to the left to lie posterior to the developing loops of small gut, where it elongates towards the diaphragm. In the left iliac fossa it normally forms a loop attached to the posterior abdominal wall by a mesentery, the sigmoid colon. With all the movement, part of the distal segment of foregut

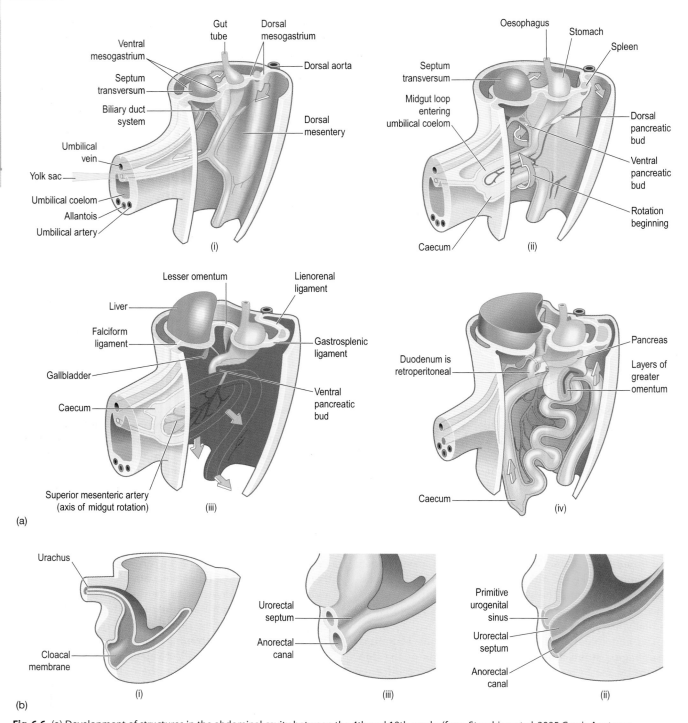

Fig. 6.6 (a) Development of structures in the abdominal cavity between the 4th and 10th weeks (from Standring et al. 2005 Gray's Anatomy 39th Edn. Churchill Livingstone, Edinburgh, with permission). (b) Division of the urogenital sinus (from Larson 2001 Human Embryology 3rd Edn. Churchill Livingstone, Philadelphia, with permission).

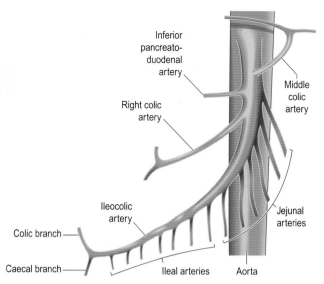

Fig. 6.32 The superior mesenteric artery and its main branches.

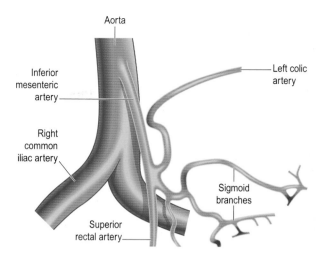

Fig. 6.33 The inferior mesenteric artery and its main branches.

arteries (Fig. 6.13) whilst on the right is found (a) the **middle colic artery** supplying the transverse colon and hepatic flexure, (b) the **inferior pancreatoduodenal artery** supplying the pancreas and third and fourth parts of duodenum, and (c) the right colic artery supplying the ascending colon from the caecum to the hepatic flexure. The terminal branch, the ileocolic artery, descends to provide an anterior and posterior caecal artery, the latter giving rise to the artery of the appendix, which must be securely ligated at appendicectomy.

The **paired renal arteries** (Fig. 6.29) pass from their origin each side of the aorta at L2 to the hilum of the right and left kidney where they may branch prior to entering the substance of the kidney. It is of note that the right renal artery is longer than the left and passes posterior to the inferior vena cava. Occasionally there may be single or multiple aberrant renal vessels passing to the lower pole of the kidney and these reflect the development of this organ.

The **inferior mesenteric artery** (Figs. 6.15, 6.33) passes caudally and to the left from its origin anterior to L3. It divides early to form (a) the **left colic artery** passing to supply the descending colon and superiorly the splenic flexure and part of the transverse colon, (b) **sigmoidal arteries** passing into the mesentery supplying the sigmoid colon, and (c) the **superior rectal artery** passing over the pelvic brim to supply the upper two-thirds of the rectum.

The **marginal artery** (Fig. 6.15) is formed by an anastomosis, along the mesenteric border and medial edges of the colon, of all colic vessels commencing with the arteries of the caecum. It is of note that the anastomosis between the superior and inferior mesenteric arteries at the splenic flexure is potentially poor, as demonstrated by the formation of ischaemic strictures at this site.

The **common iliac vessels** (Fig. 6.29) pass laterally from the bifurcation of the aorta at L4 to the right and left to divide again anterior to the sacroiliac joint. They lie slightly anterior and to the left of the common iliac veins and are separated from the small intestine by the peritoneum. On the left they are crossed by the mesentery of the sigmoid colon. At their bifurcation they lie posterior to the ureter and form the **external** and **internal iliac arteries**. The latter pass into the pelvis whilst the former pass laterally and anteriorly around the pelvic brim to leave the abdominal cavity deep to the mid-inguinal point. Just prior to passing deep to the inguinal ligament, the **inferior deep epigastric artery** arises medial to the deep inguinal ring. It then passes cranially on the peritoneal aspect of the anterior abdominal wall supplying rectus abdominis.

Other branches of the abdominal aorta

- **Adrenal arteries** arise on each side (Fig. 6.29) from the aorta itself and are short, passing straight into the adrenal glands.
- **Gonadal arteries** also arise from the aorta at L3 but these paired vessels descend obliquely towards the pelvic brim, crossing anterior to the external iliac arteries. In the male they continue anterior to the corresponding external iliac vessel before passing through the deep inguinal ring into the inguinal canal. In the female the vessels pass on to the lateral wall of the pelvic cavity. These vessels also supply the accompanying ureter, where they run together.
- The **median sacral artery** descends from the bifurcation of the aorta to supply the lower rectum and surrounding structures.
- **Spinal arteries** arise at each vertebral level as a pair of vessels passing posteriorly wrapping around each vertebral body.
- **Inferior phrenic arteries** pass upwards towards and supply the diaphragm. They also usually send a branch to supply the adrenal glands.

Venous drainage

In the abdomen, like elsewhere, the veins run alongside the corresponding arteries, draining body wall and viscera alike back to the **inferior vena cava**. This large single central vein lies to the right of midline and runs parallel to the aorta. It is formed by the union of the **common iliac veins** anterior to L5 and runs cranially on the vertebral bodies to pierce the diaphragm at T8 (Fig. 6.34). However, in the abdomen there is a major difference whereby the veins from the abdominal gastrointestinal tract all join to form the **portal vein**. This large vein, 6–8 cm long, passes in the free edge of the lesser omentum to the **porta hepatis** of the liver from where blood drains into the inferior vena cava (Fig. 6.35).

The superior mesenteric vein lies to the right of the corresponding artery and drains in a cranial direction all blood from the midgut (third part duodenum up to, and including,

the right two-thirds of the transverse colon) and passes anterior to the uncinate process of the pancreas to lie posterior to the head of the pancreas. Here it is joined from the left by the splenic vein to which the inferior mesenteric vein has drained blood from the hindgut (distal third of transverse colon up to the superior two-thirds of the rectum) to form the portal vein. Blood from the foregut structures (abdominal oesophagus up to the second part duodenum) will drain either into the splenic vein or directly into the portal vein itself. There are locations where branches of the portal vein and the systemic veins (draining directly to the inferior vena cava) come into contact (**portosystemic anastomoses**). These include all sites where the bowel is retroperitoneal, the lower oesophagus, in the lower rectum/anal canal and around the umbilicus (due to veins passing along the ligamentum teres). These potential anastomoses only opens up creating a portosystemic link in disease states where portal blood cannot drain into, or out of, the liver into the inferior vena cava, e.g. cirrhosis of the liver.

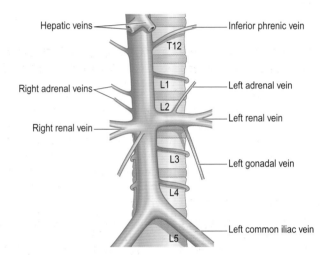

Fig. 6.34 Inferior vena cava and its main tributaries.

A 2-year-old baby girl was admitted to hospital having vomited some blood. The baby previously had an infection in the region of the umbilicus and the infection had tracked through the portal vein system and had caused portal vein thrombosis. When the girl was examined it was noted that she had enlargement of her spleen, which was easily felt in the left hypochondrium with the central notch palpable. It was also noted that she had large veins radiating out from the umbilicus (caput medusae).

These veins represent an opening up of the potential anastomoses between the systemic veins of the abdominal wall along the obliterated umbilical vein, the ligamentum teres and portal veins. In due course the bleeding was found to be coming from veins from the lower part of her oesophagus (oesophageal varices), which were injected with sclerosant to control the haemorrhage.

Renal veins pass directly from the hilum of each kidney to the inferior vena cava lying anterior to the accompanying arteries. The left vein normally lies anterior to the aorta. The **left gonadal vein** normally drains to the left renal vein, whilst the **right gonadal vein** would normally drain directly into the inferior vena cava at L2.

Adrenal veins normally pass directly to the inferior vena cava on the right and on the left to the left renal vein.

LYMPHATIC (IMMUNE) SYSTEM

Spleen

The **spleen** is a large mobile lymphoid organ, lying deep within the left hypochondrium (Fig. 6.12) within a fold of

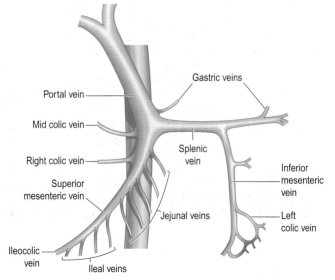

Fig. 6.35 The portal vein and main tributaries.

The female pelvis

To facilitate natural childbirth, the bony pelvis has to compromise in the female between mechanical efficiency concerning locomotion and safety in the passage of a baby through a bony ring. In the classic male pelvis the blade of the ilium is nearly vertical, giving a 'deep-sided' false pelvis, whilst the sides of the true pelvis curve inwards creating a narrow pelvic outlet (see Fig. 8.1). However, in the classic female pelvis the blade of the ilium is flatter, giving a 'shallow-sided' false pelvis, and the sides of the true bony pelvis are more vertical, opening the pelvic outlet (Figs. 7.1, 7.7). In bony terms the aim in the female pelvis is to open the canal to allow safe passage of the fetus. This is achieved by modifying the classic articulated male pelvis by:

1. lengthening of the superior pubic ramus;
2. opening of the subpubic angle (angle between both ischiopubic rami approximately 90°);
3. ischial spines more vertical;
4. opening the greater sciatic notch by increasing the angulation between the ischium and the iliac articular surface;
5. ala of the sacrum are longer than transverse diameter of the S1 vertebral body;
6. ilium articulating with fewer sacral vertebrae ($2\frac{1}{2}$ instead of 3 vertebrae).

Muscles

Muscles of the region are divided into those attaching to the inside and those gaining attachment to the outside of each innominate bone. Those attaching on the outside pass into the thigh and are considered with the lower limb. On each side of the midline (Fig. 7.8) iliacus attaches to the blade of the ilium, obturator internus attaches to the inner aspect of the obturator foramen and piriformis attaches to the anterior aspect of the sacrum. Levator ani and coccygeus pass medially from each side to form the floor or diaphragm of the pelvic cavity. Finally there are small muscles attached to the ischiopubic rami, lying in the perineum (see Fig. 7.21).

Iliacus

Attaching to the medial aspect of the ilium (see Fig. 8.18), the muscle fibres pass distally, to lie anterior to the superior pubic ramus, lateral to but accompanying **psoas**. Distally it attaches to the lesser tubercle of the femur. When active this muscle will forcibly flex the hip joint. Innervation is from the femoral nerve.

Obturator internus

This short rotator of the hip joint attaches to the bone surrounding the inner (pelvic) aspect of the obturator foramen (Fig. 7.8) and to the obturator membrane, which lies across

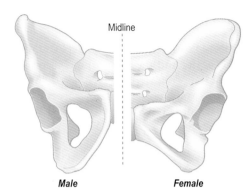

Fig. 7.7 Comparison of the main sexual differences between the male and the female pelvis.

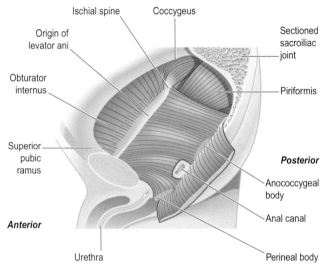

Fig. 7.8 Muscles of the pelvic walls and floor.

the foramen. The fibres pass posteriorly curving around the body of the ischium between the ischial tuberosity and the ischial spine. It then passes laterally to attach to the medial aspect of the greater trochanter of the femur. Posteriorly two small muscles join its tendon, the **gemelli**, which arise from the ischium either side of the obturator tendon (see Figs. 8.8, 8.16). When active it is a lateral rotator of the hip joint. Innervation is from the sacral plexus.

Piriformis

This triangular-shaped short rotator of the hip joint arises from the lateral aspect of the anterior surface of the sacrum (Fig. 7.8, see also Figs. 8.8, 8.15). The fibres pass laterally through the greater sciatic notch to attach to the medial aspect of the greater trochanter. It is a weak lateral rotator of the hip joint. Innervation is from the sacral plexus.

Levator ani

This thin sheet-like muscle is key to understanding the layout of the pelvic cavity and the perineum as it forms the main component of the pelvic floor (Figs. 7.8, 7.9). It gains attachment anteriorly to the posteroinferior aspect of the body of the pubis, posteriorly to the ischial spine and laterally to the fascia covering obturator internus between these two bony attachments (Figs. 7.8, 7.9). Muscle fibres pass posteriorly, medially and inferiorly to interdigitate with the fibres from the opposite side to form a midline raphe. The fibres form slings around midline structures as follows:

1. **Anterior** fibres form a sling around the urethra in the male or the vagina in the female by attaching medially to the perineal body.
2. **Middle** group of fibres form a sling around the rectoanal junction attaching anteriorly to the perineal body, the deep part of the external anal sphincter, and posteriorly to the anococcygeal body.
3. **Posterior** or lateral group of fibres. Lateral group of fibres from the fascia over obturator internus form a sling attaching to the anococcygeal body anteriorly and sacrum/coccyx posteriorly.

The levator ani:

1. supports the pelvic contents especially when intra-abdominal pressure is raised as in defaecation, micturition and parturition;
2. assists in voluntary continence of urine and faeces;
3. assists in rotating the fetus in normal childbirth.

Innervation is from the lower branches of the sacral plexus via the pudendal nerve and also directly from the sacral plexus. The anterior and middle groups of fibres are also known as pubococcygeus. Alternatively, the middle group is known collectively as puborectalis, the posterior group as iliococcygeus and the anterior group as pubovaginalis (in the female) or puboprostaticus (in the male).

Coccygeus

This small triangular muscle fills in a small defect in the pelvic floor posterior to levator ani. It passes from the ischial spine and fans out attaching to the lateral aspect of the sacrum. It supports the actions of levator ani, as it completes the muscular pelvic floor. Innervation of this small muscle is as per levator ani.

PERITONEAL CAVITY

As in the abdominal cavity, the peritoneum is reflected from the body wall on to the surface of the various structures located within the pelvic cavity, creating several key spaces or **pouches**. It is in these pouches, which differ in the male and female, that 'foreign' material (e.g. pus), if allowed, will collect. In the male the peritoneum from the posterior wall of the pelvis covers the rectum (see below), and lies on the upper surface of the pelvic diaphragm before reflecting anteriorly on the superior surface of the bladder. This pouch is known as the **rectovesical pouch** (Fig. 7.10).

However, in the female this space is divided into two by the presence of the uterus and fallopian tubes (Fig. 7.11). Therefore, as the peritoneum passes along the pelvic diaphragm from the rectum it reaches the posterior aspect of the uterus, which it covers before descending on to the anterior aspect of the uterus. From here the peritoneum continues anteriorly on to the superior surface of the bladder. Lateral to the uterus the peritoneum also passes upwards to cover the fallopian tubes to attach to the lateral pelvic wall and to the

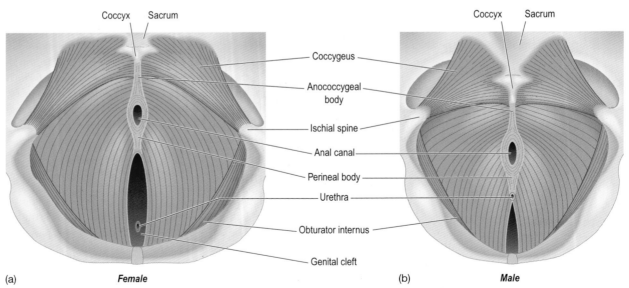

Coccyx   Sacrum   Coccyx   Sacrum

Coccygeus

Anococcygeal body

Ischial spine

Anal canal

Perineal body

Urethra

Obturator internus

Genital cleft

(a)   *Female*   (b)   *Male*

Fig. 7.9 Levator ani (viewed from below) forming most of the pelvic floor of the female and the male pelvis.

lateral aspect of the uterus, forming a peritoneal fold known as the **broad ligament**. Posteriorly the pouch between the rectum and uterus is known as the **rectouterine pouch** (of Douglas), whilst the anterior pouch between the uterus and bladder is known as the **uterovesical pouch**.

GASTROINTESTINAL SYSTEM

Rectosigmoid junction to anal sphincter

A 65-year-old man presented to his family doctor having passed bright-red blood per rectum. His doctor examined the patient rectally and noticed a hard, craggy mass located posteriorly in the lower rectum. With the examining finger it was clear that the mass was adherent to the sacrum. The patient was referred to hospital and using an endoscope a tumour was visualised and biopsied. This confirmed the diagnosis of cancer of the rectum.

The tumour was fixed and visualised radiologically (Fig. 7.12), before surgery the patient underwent a preoperative course of radiotherapy to help shrink the tumour. Subsequently at operation it was possible to remove the tumour. This involved removal of the rectum and the lower sigmoid colon was brought out as a permanent opening (colostomy) in the left lower quadrant of the abdomen.

When analysed pathologically the tumour was large, originated in the mucosa of the rectum, and had spread along the lymphatics lying alongside the superior and middle rectal vessels and into the mesorectum. At operation the surgeon had removed the mesorectum with the tumour. Unfortunately the lymph nodes along the inferior mesenteric artery and vein were involved with tumour and the patient's prognosis was poor, despite postoperative chemotherapy.

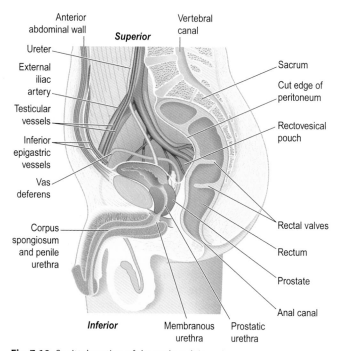

Fig. 7.10 Sagittal section of the male pelvis.

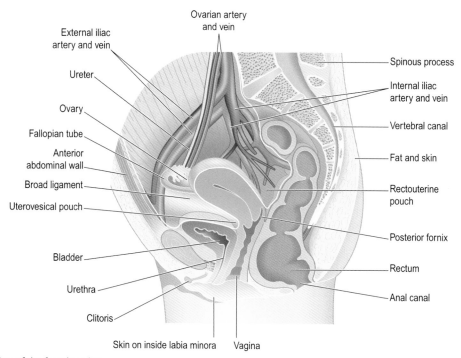

Fig. 7.11 Sagittal section of the female pelvis.

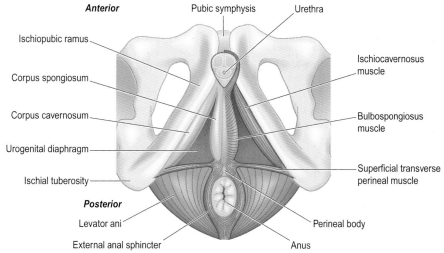

Fig. 7.24 Male urogenital triangle sectioned through the superficial perineal pouch.

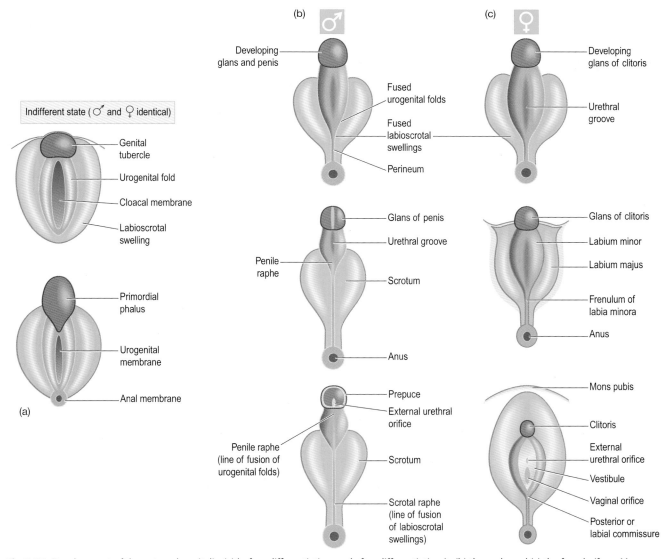

Fig. 7.25 Development of the external genitalia, (a) before differentiation, and after differentiation in (b) the male and (c) the female (from Moore Persaud 1998 The Developing Human. Saunders, Philadelphia, with permission).

Baby John was born apparently perfectly healthy, but when his mother was changing his nappy she noticed that his urine did not appear to be coming out from the end of his penis. Instead when he was passing urine it seemed to flow from the undersurface of his penis. She took the baby to his family doctor, who informed her that the baby boy had been born with *hypospadias*. The doctor explained to the mother that the baby boy, when a fetus, did not develop his penis in a normal fashion. He had incomplete fusion of the genital cleft.

The doctor referred the young boy to a paediatric surgeon who fortunately was able to perform a plastic operation to close the gap and produce a new urethra in the glans. The urethra then opened at the end of the glans in a normal external meatus. This surgery was performed as a day case and the young boy made a splendid recovery and had no further problems. Mother and baby were well pleased.

A 42-year-old woman noted a swelling on her vulva. On examination she had a 4 cm non-tender, soft cystic swelling, deep in the right labium minora posteriorly. This swelling was protruding medially and distorting the vaginal entrance (vestibule). This cystic swelling was due to a blockage of the duct of Bartholin's gland, which normally drains into the lateral side of the vagina just inside the hymen (where the vagina opens into the vestibule). These glands produce a mucoid secretion. If the duct of the gland becomes blocked, then the secretions cannot escape and they build up, gradually forming a cyst, which may develop into a very painful abscess if infection occurs. Treatment under general anaesthetic is to marsupialize (lay open) the duct. A cruciate (cross) incision was made on the vaginal aspect of the cyst and the cyst wall was sutured to the skin to create a permanent opening for gland secretions.

Hypospadias is a condition that occurs in 1 out of 250 male births and is the commonest congenital malformation of the urethra, occurring where there is incomplete fusion of both sides of the genital cleft in the male. Classically there are four types:

1. **Glandular**: here the opening of the urethra is on the underside of the glans.
2. **Coronal**: the meatus is at the junction of the glans and the shaft of the penis.
3. **Penile**: the opening is on the underside of the penile shaft.
4. **Perineal**: this is a very severe abnormality where the scrotum is split in two and does not fuse in development. This may cause confusion over the sex of the child, especially at the time of birth.

The male **corpus spongiosum** enlarges posteriorly to form the bulb of the penis and attaches securely to the superficial layer of the urogenital diaphragm. Distally it is the corpus spongiosum that will enlarge, forming the glans of the penis or clitoris. The glans is tethered to the skin covering it by a fold of mucosa, the **frenulum**, containing a small artery. In both sexes the glans is extremely well supplied with sensory nerve endings carried within the pudendal nerve. The corpora are sponge-like and with autonomic innervation (from the pelvic autonomic plexi which closes the venous drainage), and can engorge with blood, making them distend and facilitating sexual intercourse.

In the male the testes lie within the superficial pouch. However, in the female it is the **greater vestibular (Bartholin's) glands** (female equivalent of the bulbourethral glands) that lie deep to the vestibular bulb within the superficial perineal pouch. These small apocrine glands secrete into the vestibule itself.

REPRODUCTIVE SYSTEM

A 29-year-old man presented with a lump in the right testicle. This was hard and irregular. An ultrasound scan confirmed a diagnosis of a testicular tumour (Fig. 7.26). When he was 7 years old, he had an operation (orchidopexy) to bring this testicle, which was undescended, into the scrotum.

In theatre his right testicle and spermatic cord to the level of the deep inguinal ring were removed through an inguinal (groin) incision.

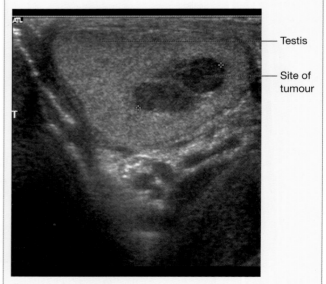

Fig. 7.26 Ultrasound image of a testicular tumour (lying between the + … +).

23 Describe the arrangement of erectile tissue in the male and female, the actions of ischiocavernosus and bulbospongiosus muscles and the relationship to the penile urethra in the male.

24 Describe the path taken by sperm in the male and the ovum in the female from their point of origin in the gonad until they leave the body.

25 Describe the general developmental pattern of the external genitalia, to allow comment on the variations that may be seen at birth.

26 Describe the main parts of the testis and the epididymis as seen in a sagittal section.

27 Describe the arteries and their main branches that supply the structures located within the pelvic cavity from the aorta and internal iliac vessels.

28 Describe the arterial supply to the pelvic gastrointestinal tract (inferior mesenteric artery, middle and inferior rectal arteries).

29 Describe the venous drainage of the pelvic gastrointestinal tract, including the portal venous system and sites of portosystemic anastomosis.

30 Discuss the principles involved in the arterial supply and venous drainage of the pelvic viscera.

31 Discuss the principles involved in the innervation of the pelvic viscera, in particular the general layout of the autonomic nerves within the pelvis.

32 Describe the pattern of lymph drainage of the pelvic organs and the implications of cancer spread.

33 Describe the lymphatic drainage of the gonads.

34 Discuss the principles involved in the innervation of the pelvic viscera.

35 Discuss the general arrangement and innervation of the perineum (anal and urogenital triangles, ischiorectal fossa) in the female and in the male.

36 Describe the pelvic course and accurately locate the femoral, obturator and sciatic nerves.

37 Describe briefly the development of the male and female gonads, commenting on their descent to their adult positions and the origin of their blood supply.

38 Describe briefly the development of the external genitalia in relation to common neonatal problems.

ASSESSMENT

Case 1

A 67-year-old presented to the A&E department at 2 a.m. with severe lower abdominal pain. He had been drinking in a pub and had not passed urine for 8 hours. On examination there was a suprapubic swelling which was tender and dull to percussion. A diagnosis of acute urinary retention was made and under aseptic conditions local anaesthetic was passed into the urethra, before a 16 ch Foley catheter was inserted into the penis.

1. Describe the path taken by the catheter as it passes into the bladder.

A rectal examination confirmed that the prostate gland was enlarged and one week later the patient was brought to theatre for transurethral resection of the prostate (TURP). A cystoscope was passed under direct vision through the urethra into the bladder, which was examined to identify the position of the ureteric orifices in relation to the bladder neck (the trigone). The cystoscope was withdrawn into the prostatic urethra and the openings of the ejaculatory ducts were noted, which must be preserved throughout the procedure.

The bladder neck or internal urinary sphincter is a ring of smooth muscle, which is closed at rest and during ejaculation. During micturition the bladder neck opens to allow urine to flow into the prostatic urethra. When the external urinary sphincter opens, micturition occurs. A TURP destroys the internal sphincter but preserves the external sphincter, which is more prominent anteriorly where it invests the urethra and lies underneath the dorsal vein complex. Thus the patient is continent but develops retrograde ejaculation following TURP. The bladder neck and prostate are then removed in 'chips' with electrocautery. A catheter is reinserted and removed when bleeding has stopped. The patient voided without difficulty. (In patients with a previous pelvic fracture, as the external sphincter is commonly damaged in the fracture, the surgeon would avoid resection of the bladder neck, as this is the only continence mechanism left.)

Case 2

A 14-year-old boy woke up in the middle of the night with very severe pain in his left testis. The pain was unbearable and he was unable to go back to sleep. He called his parents. Because the pain was so severe he was taken immediately to A&E and the doctor who examined him found that the testicle on the left side was high in the scrotum. The boy would not allow the doctor to palpate the testis because of extreme local tenderness. The doctor who examined the patient was concerned that the boy may have torsion of

ASSESSMENT *(cont'd)*

the testes. An ultrasound scan was performed, which confirmed that the testis was twisted and possibly avascular.

2. What is the blood supply to the testis?

Because of the concern that the blood supply to the testis was compromised by the twist in his spermatic cord he was taken to theatre within the hour. At operation, when the scrotum was opened the cord was found to be twisted. The testis itself was quite swollen and the cord was untwisted by the surgeon. Warm packs of saline were put over the testis to help improve its blood supply. Having untwisted the testis and with the warm surrounding packs, the blood supply improved. The surgeon was happy the testis was now viable. To prevent the twist recurring, the surgeon fixed the testis by placing sutures between the tunica vaginalis and tunica albuginea. Three sutures were inserted.

3. What is the underlying abnormality that allows this twisting to occur?

The young man went home after 24 hours. The surgeon, at outpatients 8 weeks later, felt that the left testis was a little smaller than the right. He repeated the ultrasound scan, which showed that the left testis had shrunk (become atrophic), but because it was not painful the surgeon did not take any further action.

Case 3

A 35-year-old woman undergoing childbirth had an unavoidably delayed delivery during which she spent some 8 hours trying to push the baby to be delivered vaginally. The baby was large, weighing 10 lb, and a difficult delivery ensued. Following surgery she was noticed to be very bruised and swollen around her anus and lower vaginal area and she complained to the doctor one week after the operation that she had little in the way of control of liquid faeces and at times difficulty in controlling solid faecal matter.

4. What structures might be damaged?

A defect was found in the voluntary muscle by an examining gynaecologist. She was initially offered physiotherapy and pelvic exercises which improved her incontinence only a little. In due course she underwent repair of the sphincter muscles. When examined in theatre a tear was located in the lower portion of the anal sphincter, involving both the internal anal sphincter of involuntary muscle and the lower two-thirds of the external anal sphincter of voluntary muscle. This led to an improvement in her condition, but at times, when she was having a loose stool, her incontinence would recur and she had to wear an occasional pad.

Case 4

A 60-year-old unmarried woman presented to her general practitioner with a history of increasing abdominal distension, constipation and dyspepsia. Abdominal palpation revealed a firm mass arising out of the pelvis to midway between the umbilicus and xiphisternum. The patient was referred to hospital where an MRI scan revealed a cystic and solid 30 × 20 cm mass arising from the pelvis (Fig. 7.34). There was mild left hydronephrosis and solid deposits in the region of the transverse colon.

5. What structure might be the cause of this mass?

The patient had a laparotomy, which revealed a huge tumour arising from the left ovary and a smaller one arising from the right ovary with tumour nodules growing in the greater omentum.

6. What is the blood supply to the ovary?

The left ureter was compressed by the tumour at the level of the pelvic brim, where it crossed the iliac vessels en route to the bladder. Both ovaries were excised and a hysterectomy and omentectomy performed (removal of the omentum). This was followed up by chemotherapy. Despite her widespread disease, she responded to chemotherapy and lived 4 years.

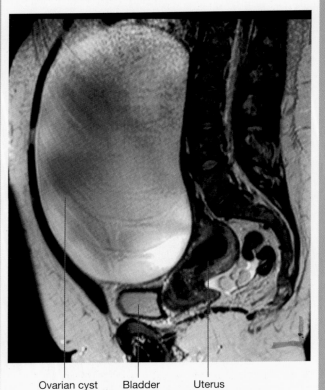

Ovarian cyst   Bladder   Uterus

Fig. 7.34 Sagittal MR scan of a large ovarian cyst.

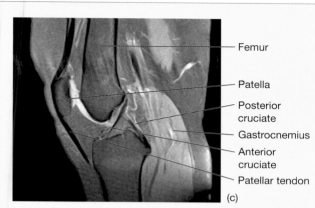

- Femur
- Patella
- Posterior cruciate
- Gastrocnemius
- Anterior cruciate
- Patellar tendon

(c)

Fig. 8.12 (*Cont'd*) Sagittal slices through a knee demonstrating a damaged anterior cruciate ligament (a and b); compare with (c) normal sagittal MR scan.

There are five key ligaments holding the femur and tibia together, the patellar, two collaterals and two cruciate ligaments (Fig. 8.11). The **patellar tendon** passes from the inferior aspect of the patella to attach to the tibial tuberosity on the superior aspect of the anterior tibial border. It is really a continuation of the quadriceps tendon (see below). The collateral ligaments lie outside the capsule separated from it by the inferior medial and lateral genicular vessels. These ligaments are designed to prevent distraction of the tibia from the femur. Laterally lies the **fibular (lateral) collateral** ligament. It is a round cord-like ligament joining the lateral femoral epicondyle to the head of the fibula and is palpable in the living knee. Medially is the broader, flatter **medial collateral** ligament. This also has a deeper layer lying deep to the medial genicular vessels, which blends with the capsule itself. It passes from the medial femoral epicondyle to the superomedial aspect of the medial tibial border. The cruciate ligaments lie within the capsule itself. They arise from the intercondylar ridge of the tibia passing cranially to attach to the femoral condyles within the intercondylar notch.

The **anterior cruciate** ligament passes from the anterior aspect of the intercondylar ridge of the tibia passing superiorly, posteriorly and laterally to attach to the medial aspect of the lateral femoral condyle. The **posterior cruciate** ligament passes from the posterior aspect of the intercondylar ridge superiorly, anteriorly and medially to the lateral aspect of the medial femoral condyle. Both ligaments are designed to prevent forward (posterior cruciate) or backward displacement (anterior cruciate) of the femur on the tibia. (*Alternatively the posterior cruciate prevents posterior movement of the tibia on the distal femur and the anterior cruciate prevents anterior movement of the tibia on the distal femur as used in testing clinically.*)

Clinically the movement of the distal tibia on the femur is tested with the knee flexed to 90°, the anterior cruciate is tested by attempting to displace the tibia anteriorly, whilst the posterior is tested by attempting to displace the tibia posteriorly. However, flexion to 20° is said to provide a more sensitive test of cruciate integrity. It has been observed that the thickened posterior capsule of the knee joint itself has a role in maintaining knee stability, supporting the role of the anterior cruciate ligament.

The patellofemoral articulation is the anterior compartment of the knee joint and allows gliding of the patella along and around the anterior aspect of the femoral condyles. Its joint space communicates with that of the tibiofemoral compartments and superiorly with the **suprapatellar bursa**, a large synovial extension of the knee joint deep to the quadriceps tendon. Because of the strength of the quadriceps muscles, if there is weakness in the pull of vastus medialis, unequal pressure is placed between the lateral patellar facet and the anterior lateral condyle (see Fig. 1.11). If prolonged and uncorrected it is a cause of anterior knee pain.

The anatomical **ankle joint** is a synovial hinge joint between the distal ends of the tibia, fibula and the superior articular surface of the talus, allowing flexion and extension. Clinically when the ankle joint is examined, the **subtalar joints** (see below) are also examined as these joints allow inversion and eversion.

The capsule of the ankle joint passes from the articular margins of the distal tibia and fibula and to the articular margins of the superior articular surface of the talus. Anteriorly the capsule extends on to the dorsal surface of the neck of the talus. Being a hinge joint there are two collateral ligaments, one medially and one laterally (Fig. 8.13). Laterally the **lateral collateral** ligament passes from the lateral malleolus dividing into three slips. The most anterior slip passes distally to the neck of the talus, the **anterior talofibular** ligament. One slip passes posteriorly to the back of the body of the talus, the **posterior talofibular** ligament. In between these two is a band passing from the lateral malleolus to the lateral aspect of the calcaneus, the **calcaneofibular** ligament. Medially the **deltoid** ligament is divided into superficial and deep layers. The superficial layer fans out from the medial malleolus anteriorly to attach to the navicular bone, the sustentaculum tali inferiorly and to the talocalcaneonavicular (or spring) ligament between these two bony points. The deep layer passes from the medial malleolus inferiorly to the medial side of the body of the talus. The muscles of the anterior (extensor) compartment, posterior (flexor) compartment and the lateral (evertor) compartment control movement at the clinical ankle joint. Inversion of the ankle is brought about from the combined action of the anterior and posterior tibialis muscles. Eversion is more limited and is brought about by the laterally placed peroneal muscles (see below).

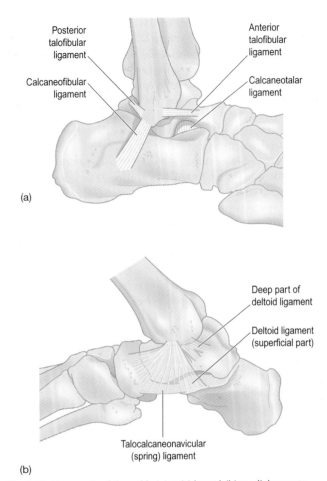

(a)

Posterior talofibular ligament

Calcaneofibular ligament

Anterior talofibular ligament

Calcaneotalar ligament

(b)

Deep part of deltoid ligament

Deltoid ligament (superficial part)

Talocalcaneonavicular (spring) ligament

Fig. 8.13 Ligaments of the ankle joint: (a) lateral, (b) medial aspects.

The many small ligaments joining adjacent tarsal and metatarsal bones maintain the **two longitudinal arches** of the foot. At rest these ligaments maintain the arches, which distribute the body weight posteriorly (proximally) on to the tubercles of the calcaneus and anteriorly (distally) on to the heads of the metatarsals. However, when moving, the short muscles of the foot and the tendons passing from the leg into the foot all provide a dynamic support to the arches, ensuring when weight is initially loaded on to the foot that the muscles are active and prevent strain of the ligaments. One key ligament in the foot is the **talocalcaneonavicular** or **spring** ligament (Fig. 8.13), passing from the sustentaculum tali of the calcaneus to the navicular bone. The superior aspect of this ligament has cartilage on its surface to provide an articular surface, completing the articular socket for the head of talus.

A 25-year-old man attended A&E one evening after injuring his right ankle. He had been jogging in a local park when he 'went over' on it, experiencing sudden pain in the lateral aspect of his right foot. On examination, the patient was tender over the lateral aspect of the foot, about three finger-

breadths anterior to the lateral malleolus. There was no evidence of a fracture on X-ray.

The clinical diagnosis was, therefore, ankle sprain, caused by a partial tear of the anterior talofibular ligament. The patient was treated by placing the foot in an elastic support bandage. The pain did settle within 2 weeks, but the patient was warned that the ankle could become painful again, if twisted within the next year.

Investing the muscles of the lower limb is the thick **deep fascia**, which forms a sleeve over the whole limb. Within this fascia, the muscles are grouped by function through thick intermuscular septa passing from the deep fascia (superficially) to the deeper bone. Within the thigh, the deep fascia is thickened laterally through the insertion of two muscles (tensor fascia lata and the upper fibres of gluteus maximus) into the fascia to form the **iliotibial band** or tract, which has a role in assisting extension and stability of the knee joint.

It is the toughness of the deep fascia in the leg that is important in ensuring the normal blood return through the muscle pump. However, occasionally it is the same toughness and lack of elasticity of the deep fascia that leads to a clinical condition, the **compartment syndrome**. In this condition there is an acute painful swelling within one or more of the muscular compartments following severe lower limb trauma. It is the structure of the deep fascia and its lack of elasticity that puts the viability of the affected tissues at risk by compressing the nerves and blood supply. Treatment involves the surgical division of the deep fascia covering the affected compartment, releasing the pressure.

In the foot the deep fascia is referred to as the **plantar aponeurosis**. This tough band passes distally from the plantar aspect of the calcaneus before dividing into five slips

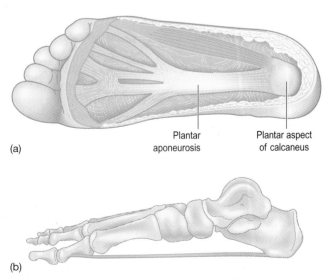

(a)

Plantar aponeurosis

Plantar aspect of calcaneus

(b)

Fig. 8.14 The plantar aponeurosis: (a) plantar and (b) medial views.

'**Toe off**' marks both the end of the stance phase and the start of swing phase for a limb. It is at this point that the hip abductors of the limb entering stance start to contract, to initiate the pull of the centre of mass towards the new stance limb. The **swing** phase starts at 'toe off' with the ankle extensors contracting to lift the toes off the ground and the hip flexors active to initiate hip flexion. With the toes now free and the limb behind the trunk, gravity pulls the limb forwards, passively flexing the hip and extending the knee joints. It is the abduction of the hip joint on the stance leg that provides the clearance for the limb as it raises the height of the hip joint of the swing leg from the ground. Through mid-swing there is little muscle activity except from the ankle extensors. Swing terminates with contraction of the hip extensors which stop the forward swing of the limb and bring about 'heel strike'.

Standing and posture

While standing upright with both feet on the ground the body can rest most of the muscles of the lower limb. In this position both knees are extended and locked, and the pelvis is pushed forwards extending the hip joint. In this posture extension of hip and knee is maintained by gravity attempting to extend these joints further and is resisted by the ligaments, allowing the muscles around each joint to relax. The ankle joint is also extended in this stance posture and as such the muscles controlling the ankle can relax. However, there is slightly increased tone in the main ankle flexors (gastrocnemius and soleus) to prevent forward sway of the limb and trunk relative to the feet. If the individual stands up on to their toes (flexed ankle), stability at the joint is achieved by balanced activity between the ankle flexors and extensors. However, when standing in high heels, the ankle extensors are not required to support the flexed ankle joint, which is supported by the shoe, though tone in the main ankle flexors will remain high.

Sitting down, standing up

When moving from the upright posture to sitting on a chair, there is a **controlled fall**. During this process the centre of body mass is normally maintained over the feet. The ankle joints are extended, the knees are unlocked and flexed and the trunk is flexed on the hip. In this position gravity is the main force increasing flexion at hip and knee and is controlled by muscle action. The **erector spinae** muscles contract to prevent further trunk flexion and maintain the centre of mass over the feet. The main muscles controlling the descent are **gluteus maximus**, contracting to slow the process of hip flexion, and the **quadriceps** controlling the degree of knee flexion. When standing up from the seated position it is the reverse; the trunk is flexed to move the centre of mass over the feet, controlled by the erector spinae, the quadriceps and gluteus maximus contract to extend the

knee and hip. As these joints extend, the erector spinae contract to bring the trunk to a more upright posture to maintain the centre of mass over the feet.

CARDIOVASCULAR SYSTEM

An 81-year-old woman slipped in her bathroom and fell. She sustained immediate pain in her left hip and was unable to get up or to weight-bear. She pressed an emergency button, which she wore around her neck. Her family found her lying on the floor and called her doctor. The doctor found her unable to weight-bear and her left leg appeared to be shortened and rotated laterally. She was taken to the hospital by ambulance. At hospital an X-ray showed that she had a fracture of the left neck of femur (Fig. 8.23a).

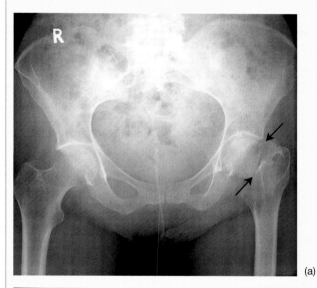

(a)

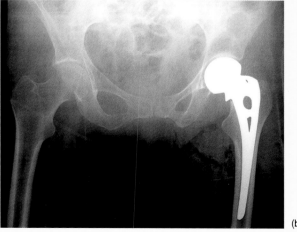

(b)

Fig. 8.23 AP radiographs of a left intracapsular fracture: (a) preoperative, (b) postoperative using a hemiarthroplasty, replacing only the femoral head.

On looking at the X-rays the orthopaedic surgeon determined that the blood supply to the head of the femur was damaged because of the position of the fracture through the neck (**subcapital**). Therefore, simply internally fixing the fracture would not be adequate as the blood supply to the head of the femur was interrupted. Subsequently, avascular necrosis and death of the head of femur would occur. Arthritis would then supervene with subsequent pain and immobility. The surgeon therefore replaced the head of the femur at operation with a prosthesis (Fig. 8.23b). The next day the patient was walking with help. She was able to go to a convalescent home after 2 weeks.

Arterial supply

Posterior to the hip joint the gluteal muscles are supplied through branches of the internal iliac artery that pass through the greater sciatic notch, the **superior gluteal artery** (lying between gluteus medius and minimus) and the **inferior gluteal artery** deep to gluteus maximus. Branches of the gluteal vessels anastomose with each other.

However, the main source of arterial blood to the lower limb lies anterior to the hip joint, as a direct continuation of the **external iliac artery**, known as the **femoral artery** (Fig. 8.24). It commences deep to the mid-inguinal point (midway between the anterior superior iliac spine and pubic symphysis), passing into the thigh within a sleeve of transversalis fascia, the femoral sheath. At this point, just distal to the inferior epigastric artery branch of the external iliac artery, it lies anterior to the tendon of psoas. The femoral artery continues distally on the medial aspect of the thigh first through a triangular space, the femoral triangle, and then a tunnel, the subsartorial canal. This artery terminates as it passes through the hiatus in adductor magnus (approx. 10 cm proximal to the adductor tubercle) when it becomes known as the **popliteal artery** and now lies posterior to the femur.

The femoral artery normally has one main branch in the femoral triangle, the **profunda femoris**, which passes

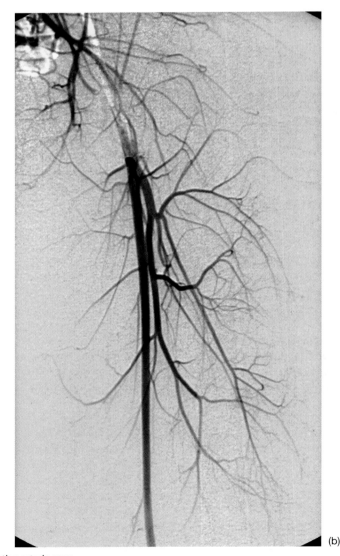

Gluteal artery

Femoral head

Femoral artery

Lateral circumflex femoral artery

Femoral artery

Superior genicular artery

External iliac artery

Medial circumflex femoral artery

Profunda femoris with perforating branches

Medial aspect of femur

(a)

(b)

Fig. 8.24 Femoral artery and its main branches: (a) diagrammatic, (b) selective arteriogram.

ASSESSMENT (cont'd)

family doctor and the local hospital frequently. Two months previously he had sustained a minor knock to his knee again.

8. Describe the compartments in the knee in which blood could collect.

On examination he had a painful reduced range of movement of his right knee.

9. What might a plain X-ray show?

An MRI scan was also performed and this confirmed quite marked degenerative changes in the knee.

10. Describe which parts of the knee joint become involved in degenerative changes.

Haemophilia is caused by deficiency of factor VIII due to an abnormal gene on the X chromosome. Males are affected and females transmit the disease and patients have an increased tendency to bleeding into joints. With repeated bleeding the joints undergo degenerative changes. He required a total knee replacement in the future, during which he would receive factor VIII replacement.

Case 4

A 76-year-old woman presented to her general practitioner complaining of vague pain in the right side of her pelvis. She was otherwise well, although 3 years previously she had a right mastectomy for breast carcinoma. At that time she had received chemotherapy and radiotherapy. Her family doctor gave her anti-inflammatory drugs and the pain settled for a while. However, one week later she sustained a very minor trip and was unable to move her right hip and right leg. She lay on the ground with the leg shortened and laterally rotated.

11. What may have caused her leg to be so painful that she could not move it?

12. Why is the leg shortened and held laterally rotated?

13. A plain X-ray was performed (Fig. 8.34). Describe what it shows.

14. Why did this lady's femoral neck fracture so easily after a minor trip?

She had a secondary deposit from her original breast cancer, which had weakened the bone in the region of the femoral neck. Breast cancer has a tendency to spread to liver, bones and lung. She had the femoral neck pinned and was referred to Oncology for palliative care.

15. Describe the incisions that the surgeon may have to make to get access to the femoral neck and which muscles he may have to cut.

Following pinning of the hip she required postoperative radiotherapy and was comfortable for the remaining 6 months of her life. She could walk with help.

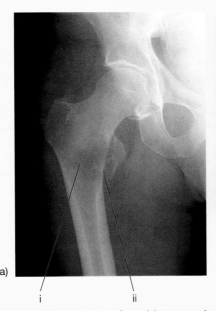

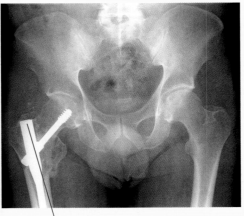

Internal fixation to reduce fracture

(a)

(b)

i   ii

Fig. 8.34 X-ray of the right femur in case 4 above: (a) preoperative, (b) postoperative demonstrating internal fixation.

ANSWERS

1. Femoral pulse at the midpoint of the inguinal line (halfway between the anterior superior spine and the pubic symphysis). Popliteal artery in the popliteal fossa with firm pressure against the distal part of the femur. Dorsalis pedis artery (normally felt between the tendons of extensor hallucis longus and extensor digitorum longus on the dorsum of the foot). Posterior tibial artery, posterior to the medial malleolus.

2. (a) Aorta, (b) femoral artery, (c) common iliac artery, (d) internal iliac artery, (e) renal arteries.

3. One would expect the internal iliac artery to provide an increased flow through the inferior gluteal and possibly the superior gluteal arteries. These would provide blood flow within the cruciate anastomosis with a retrograde flow of blood passing into the two circumflex femoral vessels, and the profunda femoris through the perforating arteries.

4. When harvesting the great saphenous vein, the four main tributaries at the level of the saphenofemoral junction must be securely ligated. Then before using the vein it must be reversed so that the distal end of the vein is attached to the femoral artery proximal to the blockage. This will ensure that the venous valves become non-functional as the new arterial blood flow will follow the normal flow of blood through the vessel.

5. The thigh is innervated by the femoral nerve anteriorly, the obturator nerve medially and the sciatic nerve posteriorly. The leg and foot muscles are innervated by the sciatic nerve.

6. With a laceration to the posterior thigh, integrity of the sciatic nerve is in question. The femoral and obturator nerves should be functioning normally. On examination, if the sciatic nerve was totally sectioned there would be complete paralysis of the hamstring muscles of her thigh, and of all muscles distal to the knee. Cutaneous sensation would be absent on the posterior aspect of the calf, distal third of the leg, and dorsum and sole of the foot. There would be a noticeable lack of voluntary movement of the foot and ankle, while the knee could be extended though not flexed voluntarily.

7. She would require a splint to stabilise the right foot and ankle, maintaining them in a neutral position. There should be no problem with knee extension, so she would develop a gait pattern which involved keeping the right knee joint in the extended position, especially at heel strike. The swing phase on the right would most likely be shortened to reduce the strain on the knee extensors at, and immediately after, heel strike. Hip extension should still be intact through reliance on gluteus maximus, as

the hamstrings would be non-functional. In addition she would most likely require a crutch to provide support and confidence in the limb.

8. The blood usually collects in the joint between the condyles of the femur and tibial plateau surrounding the cruciate ligaments, but it can extend into the suprapatellar bursa (between the lower femoral shaft and the quadriceps). Posteriorly the joint space communicates with synovial spaces, 'bursae', deep to the medial head of gastrocnemius and beneath semimembranosus, which may fill with blood.

9. There might be evidence of damage to the articular surfaces with osteophyte formation (extra bone) (Fig. 8.35).

10. The tibial plateau and femoral condyles.

11. She may have sustained a fracture of the femoral neck.

12. Freed from the restraints imposed by the normal neck and head of femur, following a fracture of the femoral neck, the gluteal muscles contract and draw the greater trochanter proximally. Freed from the restrictions imposed by the normal hip joint itself, psoas and iliacus attached to the lesser trochanter are now free to draw it anteriorly, causing lateral rotation of the shaft of the femur. For the same reason the adductors attaching posteriorly to the linea aspera are free to laterally rotate the femur rather than their usual action of medial rotation.

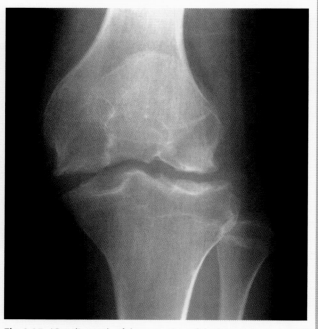

Fig. 8.35 AP radiograph of degeneration of the knee joint as a result of recurrent bleeds into the joint space.